The
Art *of*
Bathing

*For Lai Lin and
Alfie, naturally.*

Ophelia Wellspring is the pen-name of an author
and editor who lives with their partner, two children,
and a dog, not far from the sea.

Important: Aromatherapy and meditation can help with all manner of physical ailments, but this book is not intended as an alternative to personal medical advice. Aromatherapy oils are highly concentrated. The reader should follow the instructions on the packaging of selected products to ensure the oils are being used safely and effectively. Any readers who are pregnant or have a compromised immune system should consult a healthcare practitioner before use. The reader should consult their doctor about any symptoms that may require diagnosis or medical attention. While the advice and information in this book are believed to be accurate, neither the author nor publisher can accept any legal responsibility or liability for any omissions or errors herein.

OPHELIA
WELLSPRING

The Art *of* Bathing

Red Wheel

CONTENTS

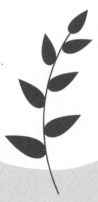

H ow often have you longed to drop everything and head off for a spa retreat? To take a healing break, find a moment to recharge your batteries, and—most importantly—seize a rare chance to put yourself first? If you're like me, you find yourself torn between the demands of work and family, with time and money constantly stretched, and there often seems to be nothing we can do about it. We feel a little like caged hamsters, constantly spinning a wheel, never stopping, yet never seeming to get anywhere, either.

Fortunately for us, the answer is sitting right there in the corner of the bathroom. Used wisely, the humble tub can become a revitalizing home spa that is more effective than you ever suspected possible. It will be a refuge from the stresses and strains of the world, and the place where you can go to re-energize. All you need is a half hour, a few essential oils, and this book.

You'll find that the combination of water, aromatherapy, meditation, and music has an incredible power to restore. You'll gain mental energy, you'll improve your physical condition, and, most importantly, you'll enjoy more positive emotions.

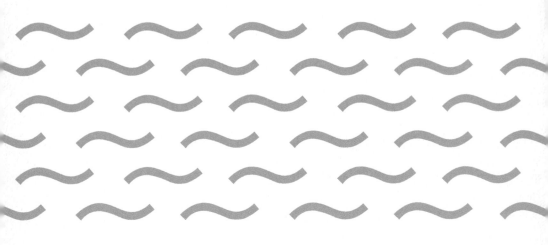

Even better, it's cheap! Essential oils aren't expensive to buy in the quantities you need for an aromatic bath, and you can build up your healthful collection over time, picking up bottles one by one.

Each treatment in this book includes an aromatherapy mix and a focused meditation aimed at a particular need. There's also an introduction to the amazing world of essential oils, and you'll learn how water, music, and meditation also play their own healing roles—so when you step into that steaming tub, you'll know exactly what's going on in your mind, body, and soul.

Over time you'll become an expert on home spa treatments, and will no doubt come up with your own essential-oil blends. Meanwhile, you'll discover that the priceless benefits of meditation become more and more powerful with regular practice, whether you practice as part of a bathtime treatment or any other time. Literally hundreds of studies now show that it's one of the best ways to keep your life on a happier, healthier, more productive path.

So I hope that this nourishing time in that humble bathtub becomes a regular part of your life, just as it is mine.

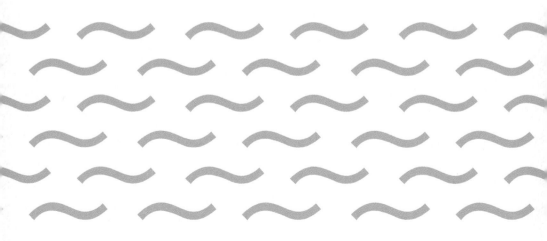

THE POWER OF WATER

Whether it's the bath, the pool, a lake, or the open ocean, there is something about water that attracts us in a completely primal way. We love to float, to let the water take our weight, and simply feel it lap against our skin: a sensory immersion, it relaxes us, frees us from tension, and warms or cools us deliciously.

Some evolutionary biologists have hypothesized that at some point in the history of our species, humans were semi-aquatic, spending much of our time swimming and finding food underwater—which could account for the fact that we have so much less hair on our bodies than our nearest relations—other primates like chimps and gorillas. While this idea is controversial, it might also explain why we love spending time in, around, and on water as much as we do. Most primates avoid deep water: humans seek it out. We pay more to live in places with a sea view, we travel long distances to take vacations on the beach, and we love sailing, swimming, diving, and all manner of other pastimes that bring us into closer contact with it. Is this because it is our natural environment?

Since classical times, when the Romans, Egyptians, and Greeks built bath-houses with a mixture of cold- and warm-water pools, we have known of the benefits of balneotherapy—the practice of using baths for relaxation and psychological well-being. Indeed, when they discovered natural hot springs they usually built a temple nearby. Hippocrates, who lived in Greece 2,500 years ago and is still widely called the "father of medicine," researched the effects of hot and cold baths on the human body, and the popularity of bath-houses in the classical world owed much to his thinking. His contemporaries used sulfurous springs to treat skin conditions and muscular and joint pain. But it wasn't just the Greeks and Romans: cultures around the world, from Japan to Aztec Mexico, had their own distinctive takes on the bath-house, and bathing has now been scientifically proven to elevate your mood, improve your sleep, relieve muscle pain, reduce blood pressure, relieve cold and flu symptoms, soothe irritated skin, and improve your alertness. There is even evidence that, by stimulating the circulation and raising your heart rate, a warm bath burns as many calories as a brisk walk! All of these individual benefits will add up to a real difference to your sense of general well-being, a reduction in stress, and—long-term—better health.

For a bath to boost your cardiovascular system and help your physical health, it should raise your core body temperature by about one degree Fahrenheit (or half a degree Celsius), so the water doesn't need to be overly hot—certainly it should be easy to climb into. That's enough to get the blood flowing faster, and give your heart the easiest workout ever. Skin flushes in a hot bath, by the way, for the same reason that it does when you walk fast on a hot day. Your body feels itself overheating and sends blood rushing to the surface to cool it down. In warm air, this works well, but if you are in a bath that's slightly warmer than your body temperature (most people find a temperature of 100°F/38°C comfortable) it has the opposite effect: the extra blood warms up and carries the heat back to your core.

Hot baths affect our skin, too; at more than 112°F (44°C) the water will melt away the natural moisturizers that sit on the surface of our skin. This affects older people more: so the piping-hot bath that you enjoyed at twenty years old may leave your skin dried-out and feeling itchy after you've turned forty. Something between 104 and 109°F (40 and 43°C) should be comfortable—hot, but not painful. If you want to hit a specific temperature, use a floating thermometer (you can get them at baby supply stores) to make sure your bath is perfect every time.

The stress-relieving qualities of a warm bath are harder to measure—although we all know them to be real. Mental stress, in the long term, is terrible for your health, causing inflammation in the body and making you more susceptible to illness as well as muscular tensions and pains. These physical symptoms, as well as sleeplessness, are all problems that will have a massive effect on your quality of life: but don't worry, with the simple guidelines in this book you will be able to alleviate them and enjoy better days and nights.

All that said, we should be careful not to confuse balneotherapy with hydrotherapy, the medical field of using water to regulate body temperature, and to aid recovery from burns or muscle injury. The wellness benefits of balneotherapy are real, but the medicinal claims that expensive spa resorts often make don't always stack up, so you should have realistic expectations of what bathing can do for you, and if serious pain or other symptoms persist, you should, of course, consult your doctor.

There's one question that you're probably keen to know the answer to: why, exactly, do our fingers and toes wrinkle up when they've been in the water for a while? For many years it was thought that water was passing through the skin and into the flesh: but researchers learned in the 1930s that it's caused by blood vessels contracting beneath the skin, and it doesn't happen when there is nerve damage in the fingers. This suggests that it is an involuntary reaction from the body's autonomic nervous system—which also controls breathing, sweating, and our heartbeat. Why? The answer came in 2013, when a study found that wrinkled fingertips help us to pick up wet objects. By acting like the pattern on car tires, they give us added grip. Handy when you're holding on to the soap! So if you notice your fingers and toes wrinkling up, don't worry, it's not your body telling you to get out—you can stay in the tub as long as you like.

INTRODUCING ESSENTIAL OILS & AROMATHERAPY

It's a sad fact that many people are still skeptical about the benefits of aromatherapy and natural essential oils. We take it for granted that some plants sting us painfully, that others contain the vitamins that we need to survive, that coffee beans stimulate us, and that certain mushrooms and cacti make us vividly hallucinate; why then is it so hard to accept that other plants, like bergamot, rosemary, or orange, contain natural chemicals that are, in their own ways, every bit as powerful?

The moment I realized this power for myself was shortly after I burned my hand while cooking. Touching a hot grill, I found myself grimacing with pain, and when one of my guests told me to apply Lavender oil, I was skeptical and only agreed out of good manners. To my complete surprise, a tiny drop not only relieved the pain but also allowed the skin to rapidly heal itself. The next day, where I had expected to see an ugly scar or blister, there was only a painless red blush and the day after that, nothing. I can't think of any other cure for a burn that works so well. And that is only one of Lavender's uses: it will also relieve headaches, repel mosquitos, and disinfect a graze.

Inspired by this discovery, I started looking at the healing properties of other natural compounds, and I was amazed to find that literally hundreds of plants yield essential oils that can help our health and happiness. Many of them have already found their way into mainstream medicines: for instance, Peppermint oil is widely prescribed as a treatment for Irritable Bowel Syndrome (IBS).

But unlike synthetic, laboratory-derived drugs, essential oils rarely cause side-effects, and they pass through our body without leaving any trace. They are also usually applied more efficiently than conventional pharmaceuticals, as we don't swallow them, forcing them to mix with the fiery acids in our stomach or the powerful bacteria in our gut. Instead, we inhale them or apply them to the skin, where they are absorbed directly into our system. This means that even tiny amounts of the active chemicals smartly bring powerful benefits.

Each essential oil contains a mixture of many active compounds, from chemical families like esters, terpenes, ketones, alcohols, aldehydes, and phenols. Don't be intimidated by these technical terms; many of these organic chemicals are related to the amino acids that are the building blocks of every cell in our body. We respond well to essential oils because the compounds that they deliver are so close to the compounds that our bodies produce. That's probably why we instinctively find their aromas so delightful. Our noses recognize their potential benefits and encourage us to spend time with them!

But where should you begin? You are unique, with your own burden of aches, pains, stresses, and strains, so how do you work out which of the hundreds of essential oils out there are the right ones to lighten your load?

HOW TO CHOOSE YOUR ESSENTIAL OILS

The easiest way to use this book is to pick a treatment that meets your needs, obtain the few essential oils that it calls for, and drop them as directed into a warm bath. With just a little thought, though, you can start creating your own mixtures using the oils introduced below. There's a brief description of the physical and mental ailments for which each can be effective, so it's simple to work out where to start.

Nearly all essential oils pass through the body without leaving a trace, and their effects don't last long, so if you want to use them for any chronic conditions, or regular stressful feelings, then build them into your daily routine. Happily, it is nearly impossible to do any harm with essential oils in small doses. The worst that can usually happen is that a remedy doesn't work as well as you'd hoped, in which case, vary the treatment and find a different oil that does. The important exception is pregnancy: expectant mothers should take care to double-check that any oil they use is safe for them. Some essential oils are best used in small doses, and these are flagged up in this book. Otherwise, if you feel like adding a drop or two more or less to suit your own preferences, then go right ahead.

Important: Essential oils should always be kept out of the reach of small children and pets. In particular, make sure that your cat or dog doesn't have the opportunity to lick at anything containing Peppermint, Eucalyptus, Tea Tree, or Ylang Ylang oils, or any citrus oils like Lemon or Grapefruit.

Aromatherapy is a complicated art, with ancient roots in cultures around the world, and although there is now plenty of sound medical evidence that essential-oil remedies work on everything from burns to emotional stress (and we know the compounds that each consists of), we know less about exactly how they react with the chemistry of our bodies. So any account of essential oils and their uses is based more on the hands-on experience of practitioners— and the folk wisdom of generations—than controlled, double-blind laboratory trials. For this reason, sources do occasionally disagree with each other, especially online. Although this list has been compiled using multiple references (for more details, see the Further Reading section on page 140), you should not view it as definitive or exhaustive, but as a sensible starting point for your own journey into aromatherapy. Over time, you'll discover which essential oils work particularly well for you, and you can build up your own repertoire. Finally, make sure that you get your oils from a reputable source. Be suspicious of anywhere that prices every oil equally—and make sure that oils are freshly manufactured and well packaged.

There are something like three hundred essential oils available, so the range on offer can seem baffling and intimidating. With this handy guide to all of the oils that are mentioned in this book you'll be able to work out which will be the most useful to you. This list first summarizes physical, then mental effects.

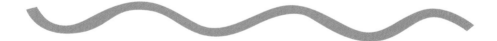

🌢 *Basil*
A stimulating tonic that helps the body cleanse itself and brings energy to your mind: good for awakening, alertness, and focus.

🌢 *Bergamot*
The sunniest of all essential oils, this is great for the skin and urinary tract; it is also a useful anti-depressant, bringing confidence and contentment.

🌢 *Black Pepper*
Stimulates and calms the digestion, and is generally fortifying; psychologically, it brings a powerful warmth, with reconnective and sometimes aphrodisiac qualities. Don't use more than three drops in the bath.

🌢 *Cardamom* (or Cardamon)
Great for the digestion, stimulating the appetite, and for the respiratory tract: it also lifts the spirits, inspires courage, and reduces worry.

🌢 *Cedarwood (Atlas)*
Useful for the nose, throat, and lungs, this is strongly antiseptic and also increases confidence and reduces fear. It helps with meditating, too. Virginian Cedarwood is similar, but has less potent effects: use Atlas Cedarwood, if you can.

🌢 *Chamomile Roman*
(or Roman Chamomile)
One of the key essential oils, this reduces inflammation in the body, so it's great for the skin and the soft tissues, and it calms the mind, too. Do not confuse with German or Moroccan Chamomile, which have different effects.

🌢 *Clary Sage*
This calms the body, so it's useful for PMS and insomnia, and it relaxes your muscles. Deeply relaxing, useful for meditation, it also lifts your soul.

🌢 *Coriander*
Boosts the appetite, and lifts the spirits, so it is particularly useful if you are convalescing or getting over an injury.

🌢 *Cypress*
Strongly astringent, this helps with circulatory problems, but it is included here more for the strength it brings to your soul.

🌢 *Eucalyptus* (or Eucalyptus Blue Gum: Lemon-Scented Eucalyptus is similar). Helping you breathe freely and clearly, this is used for coughs, colds, bronchitis, and catarrh: it also clears the mind, bringing a sense of freedom and potential.

🌢 *Frankincense*
Helps with some skin conditions, and is one of the most spiritual oils. A natural partner to meditation, this helps you breathe steadily and calmly, reducing stress and fortifying the soul.

🜄 *Geranium* (or Rose Geranium)
Regulates and balances hormones, making it useful for PMS and other life changes: it has a similar effect on our moods and mind, restoring you to an even keel.

🜄 *Ginger*
Never use more than three drops of Ginger in your bath—it's highly stimulating. Useful for the circulation and digestion, and against the cold. Mentally, it is good for introspection, self-awareness, and understanding your place in the world.

🜄 *Grapefruit*
Useful for hangovers and other times that you need to clear your system: but mood-boosting, spirit-lifting, clarity-bringing Grapefruit is mainly useful for its considerable psychological benefits.

🜄 *Jasmine*
Warning—this oil is expensive! But you only need small amounts of it. Useful for the female reproductive system, it reduces tension, boosts mood, helps with period pain, and may be an aphrodisiac.

🜄 *Juniper*
Cleans and purifies the blood, and is also helpful for cystitis and other urinary tract infections. It has a similar effect on the mind, clearing it and driving out negative emotions.

🜄 *Lavender*
Healing burns, lowering blood pressure, helping you sleep, and much more, this is one of the truly "essential" essential oils. It's also useful against worry and fear, irritability, and panic. Get yourself a large bottle!

🜄 *Lemon*
Another incredibly versatile oil, Lemon always restores balance and refreshes body and mind. It reduces nausea, helps your digestion, and lifts your mood. Don't use too much in a bath: three drops is enough.

🜄 *Lemongrass*
Works well on muscular aches and the soft connective tissues; brings mental energy and focus, aiding concentration.

🌢 *Marjoram*
Relaxes tight muscles and comforts
a troubled mind.

🌢 *Neroli*, see Orange Blossom

🌢 *Nutmeg*
Good for muscular aches and
pains, this will also calm you,
and inspire imaginative leaps
and creative breakthroughs.

🌢 *Orange* (or Sweet Orange)
A good all-round mood booster, this
has similar physical effects to its cousin,
Lemon: it restores balance and helps
to smooth out an uneven or painful
digestion. To our minds, it brings
optimism, energy, and openness.

🌢 *Orange Blossom* (or Neroli)
Expensive: it's useful for diarrhea
and insomnia, but it is included here
for its aphrodisiac qualities, which
you may find worth the price!

🌢 *Peppermint*
Stimulates your mind, boosts your
memory, relieves gas and arthritis.
Included in this list as it is one of the
most common and useful essential
oils, but some find that it can irritate

the skin, so it is not used in any of this
book's spa treatments. Put a couple of
drops onto a cloth and inhale it, or use
it in a candle with Eucalyptus instead.

🌢 *Rose Otto*
One of the jewels in the aromatherapist's crown, this works well for
headaches, PMS, and migraines—and
for treating many kinds of sadness,
from bereavement to regret or remorse.

MY FIVE "ESSENTIAL" ESSENTIAL OILS

The best way to start
an argument between
aromatherapists is to define
a short list of "essential"
essential oils. There are so
many useful oils, with so
many different applications,
that it really is a fool's errand.
But, in writing this book, I've
found myself turning to five
oils in particular. For your
information—and to disagree
with!—they are Chamomile
Roman, Geranium, Lavender,
Lemon, and Rosemary.

◆ *Rosemary*

This stimulates body and mind alike and is another essential oil that everyone should have in their home. Great for muscular aches and injuries, reducing pain, and enhancing brainpower and memory.

◆ *Sandalwood*

An unusually thick, viscous oil. Effective for a sore throat, the skin, and bronchitis, sandalwood is also useful for anyone who needs to find their voice and express themselves. This may be the cause of its powerful aphrodisiac qualities!

◆ *Tea Tree* (or Ti-Tree)

Strong antiseptic and antimicrobial properties make this a good oil for fighting off infection or illness: it also inspires confidence. The smell is medicinal, though, and not for everyone.

◆ *Vetiver*

Known as the "oil of tranquility," Vetiver brings balance, and is recommended for menopause and other points of change. It's also deeply relaxing and meditative.

◆ *Ylang Ylang*

Lowers blood pressure, and therefore anxiety and panic. Only small amounts are necessary: experts often blend it with a citrus-based oil like Lemon or Bergamot.

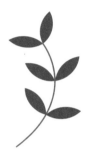

Important: If you have a dog, be considerate—its sensitive nose will find a bathroom steaming with powerful essential oils to be somewhat overwhelming, and particular oils can be harmful to pets either in large amounts or if consumed! Put your pooch somewhere well ventilated during your treatment. The same may apply to your cat.

HOW TO BLEND ESSENTIAL OILS

One of aromatherapy's many joys is that anyone can start making their own blends once you have two or more oils. A basic reference to the oils' properties will start you off—as will an internet search—and many people find that this works well for them. If you want to take a more scientific approach, then Rosemary Caddy's *Essential Blending Guide* breaks down the chemical composition of each oil and allows you to be completely systematic about making your blends, balancing esters with monoterpenes, sesquiterpenes with ketones, and so on.

HOW TO APPLY YOUR ESSENTIAL OILS

The shops are full of bath salts, bath oils, bubble baths, and scented candles, and it can be hard to know which way works best, or indeed if any way is better than another. The good news is that all of these different delivery methods are effective, and with a little thought it's easy to choose the right one for you. Just decide which oils you need (there are many remedies in the second part of this book) and apply them in the correct proportions, following the instructions given.

DROPPING DIRECTLY

This is the simplest way to inhale a rich mixture of essential oils and get them to work from the inside out. Run a warm bath, with no bubble bath or other additions, and keep the bathroom door closed so the steam doesn't dissipate. Add five to ten drops of essential oils, in the proportions specified, and sink into the water. Inhale deeply and slowly through your nose.

The volatile oils will jump off the surface and hover just above it—exactly where you'll be breathing in. Inhaling through your nose is more effective than through your mouth, as it rushes the oils' powerful compounds over the sensitive, absorbent tissues of your olfactory epithelium—which has a hotline to your brain.

BATH CRYSTALS

It's easy to make your own bath crystals that combine the benefits of aromatherapy and a warm salt soak, which diffuses the essential oils so they are absorbed through your skin. Crush up about 9oz (250g) of washing soda (sodium carbonate) crystals, add a total of twenty drops of essential oils (in the correct proportions) and mix thoroughly.

Keep the crystals in a dark glass (not plastic) jar, in a cool place away from direct sunlight. That jar will give you enough salts for two baths. If you want to color-code your crystals, or simply add a little tone to your home spa, then you can dye the crystals with a couple of drops of food coloring.

BATH OILS

If you suffer from dry skin, then a long, hot bath may leave you feeling less comfortable than before. In that case, try a cooler temperature, and use a bath oil as a base for your own essential oil remedy.

You need an unscented dispersible bath oil base, which consists of a light vegetable oil (often almond oil) and a small amount of emulsifier that allows the oil to mix into the bathwater and not float on the surface. These typically come in bottles of 2fl oz or 4fl oz (50ml or 100ml): add fifty drops of essential oil, in the correct proportions, to a smaller bottle, one hundred drops to a larger one. Shake vigorously to disperse the essential oils through the bath oil base, and store in a cool, dark place.

To use, run the bath, then add about 10ml (two teaspoons) of your mixture to the hot water, and mix it around. The bath oil turns cloudy on contact with water, but that's nothing to worry about.

CANDLES

Nothing relaxes us more than candlelight gleaming through the steam rising off a hot tub, and it gets even better when the candle's flame also diffuses essential oils. You have to be careful, though, to make sure that the flame doesn't burn off the oils before they have a chance to work their magic. So you always need a fat candle, which melts to give a wide puddle of hot wax for the oils to evaporate from. If you are adding essential oils to a plain, unscented candle, light it some time in advance, wait for the top to liquefy, and add your essential oils as far from the candle's flame as possible. You only need a small amount—6–8 drops is usually about right, depending on the proportions that your remedy demands and the size of your bathroom.

If you are confident that you will return to the same remedy time and again, then it's worth taking the time to make your own candles. These use a lot of essential oils, so it can be a significant investment, but it more than pays off over time as you access your personal remedy as easily as striking a match.

You'll need:
- a soy wax candle-making kit, including cotton wicks

- an old teacup or candle holder

- 50 drops of your chosen essential oils, in the correct proportion

Follow the kit instructions to melt the candle wax (you need to take care with the temperature, otherwise the candle will not set smoothly), shake the essential oils into the bottom of the teacup, then gently pour in just under 1 cup (225ml) of molten wax. Stir carefully with a chopstick to ensure that the oils are evenly distributed through the wax, then drop in your wick and allow to cool. Before use, trim the wick so that only ½ inch (1cm) protrudes above the surface of the solid wax.

Light the candle five or ten minutes before you run the bath, and leave it in the bathroom with the door closed. When the tub's full, turn the lights off, slide into the hot water, and enjoy the warm glow of the flame's reflections.

HOMEMADE BUBBLE BATH

If, like me, you enjoy idly playing with bubbles as they float around the surface of the tub, yet don't like the harsh synthetic odors of their artificial fragrances, don't worry! You can easily make your own unique bubble bath, which gives you all of the fun and all of the benefits of natural essential oils. An added benefit is that homemade bubble baths, unlike nearly all products you see in store, don't contain sodium lauryl sulfate, a bubbling agent that can irritate sensitive skin.

To make your own bubble bath, you need:

– 1 cup (250ml) of spring water or distilled water (or, if it's all you have, tap water that has been boiled then allowed to cool)

– 1 cup (250ml) of liquid castile soap (this is vegetable-based and vegan-friendly)

– ½ cup (125ml) of vegetable glycerin

– 40 drops of your chosen essential oils, in the correct proportions

Thoroughly mix the water, soap, and glycerin (which has a tendency to sink to the bottom of the mixture if you let it) to make an even solution. Add the essential oils, and mix thoroughly again to ensure that they are evenly distributed. Bottle in dark glass, if possible, and keep in a cool, dark place. This recipe gives you enough for four baths. Just add a quarter of your bubble bath as the bath runs and watch the scented bubbles go crazy!

HEATED DIFFUSER

Warming up the essential oils so that they vaporize, these use an oil burner or candle flame to heat a small bowl. A few drops—no more than ten—in the bowl will diffuse quickly into the air. Light it a couple of minutes before you get into the bath and make sure the bathroom door is closed to get the full effect.

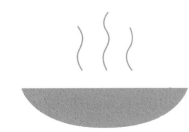

LIGHT LEVELS & RELAXATION

If you're taking your bath in the evening, then it's important—and easy—to get the lighting right. Our bodies and brains, which evolved well before the lightbulb was invented—let alone the OLED screen of your cell phone—depend on daylight, and a powerful system of hormones that affect how we feel. As the sun goes down, our bodies create high levels of the hormone melatonin, which encourages deep and restful sleep—and which in turn is essential for our brain's health. Come the dawn, our bodies create cortisol, which makes us alert and ready for the day.

Problems arise when artificial sources of light mimic the sun's rays and raise levels of cortisol in the evenings. We're stressed, we don't sleep properly, and our digestive system is thrown out of synch too.

As the spa treatments in this book are designed to return your body and mind to balance, it makes no sense to counter their effects with badly timed cortisol. So in order to benefit from the treatments in this book, you should keep light levels in your bathroom subdued. The easiest way to do that is, of course, to light a couple of candles!

MEDITATION & MINDFULNESS

Every bath-time treatment in this book has its own new meditation. A bath can powerfully restore your body, especially when you combine it with the right essential oils, but nothing is better for the mind or soul than a quiet, centering session of mindfulness or mental focus. Comfortable, still, and quiet, a bath is the perfect place to slow your breathing and reconnect with yourself.

MINDFULNESS

Mindfulness is an ancient practice, influenced by the teachings of the Buddha, who was born some 2,500 years ago, but western science has only recently caught up with it and confirmed its benefits. By helping us to understand how our minds work, and the role that our emotions play in our lives, it lets us overcome anger, anxiety, dissatisfaction, impatience, and many of the other mental habits that stop us from living fulfilled lives.

The process is simple. You nearly always start by controlling, and focusing on, your breaths. This relaxes you, and naturally tunes you in to the state of your body. Most of the meditations in this book then include a mindfulness scan, a simple way for you to pay attention to every part of your body in turn. By doing that you acknowledge the reality of the present moment: this gives you a calm, centered place from which to observe your mind, and recognize each thought that arises without judgment. Whenever you find your thoughts wandering, simply notice them, and bring your attention back to your breath. By observing

Mindfulness improves our mental well-being by helping us to lead a happy, satisfied life

emotions and feelings, we separate them from our thoughts—and, if they are destructive, take away much of their power to cause us pain. Finally, we appreciate the present moment, feeling at peace with ourselves and our surroundings.

Most people, once they have started mindful meditation, carry on and make it a regular part of their routine. Why? What does it do for them? In recent years many researchers have been looking at meditation's effects, and we now have plenty of hard evidence of its benefits.

Firstly, mindfulness improves our mental well-being by helping us to lead a happy, satisfied life. We enjoy the good things in life more, and we are more resilient when times are tough. A focus on the "here and now" means that we regret less about the past and worry less about the future; it also helps us to understand what really matters in life, and to form deeper connections with our loved ones, family, and friends. Instead of being ruled by our emotions, we can be aware of them, and see how fleeting and transitory they are.

It's also great for our physical health. Many of us quickly notice that it reduces stress levels, which it does by lowering levels of the hormone cortisol, and this in turn has huge benefits. Our hearts become healthier, our blood pressure falls, chronic pain diminishes, we sleep better, and many of us even digest our meals better. If mindfulness was a pill, every doctor in the world would prescribe it.

Finally, mindfulness helps our mental health. More and more psychotherapists use mindfulness meditation to successfully treat problems like anxiety, depression, addictions, eating disorders, and obsessive-compulsive disorder. It seems to work by helping people to accept painful emotions and experiences, rather than react to them with aversion or avoidance. Burying or denying negative emotions or memories can cause us huge problems: mindfulness is one way to acknowledge them, without judgment, thereby removing their destructive power. Plus, unlike most psychoactive medications, meditation has no negative side-effects, it's cheap, and anyone can do it.

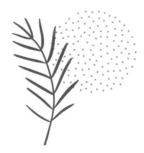

VISUALIZATION

Some of the spa treatments, especially those that are focused on some future goal, employ visualization techniques, in which you imagine a successful future and the steps you have to take to reach it. Strange as it may seem, this kind of imagining has a powerful positive effect, which has been measured in many different circumstances. It's likely that your favorite sporting star visualizes their success, for instance, but it can also help students, professionals… anyone, in fact, who's facing some kind of challenge.

CHANTING & MANTRAS

A couple of the meditations in this book use this technique, which can—if you don't come from a Buddhist or Hindu tradition—seem somewhat uncomfortable. By repeating a word, we encourage ourselves to contemplate its meaning, and this repetition can also clear our minds just as breathing meditations do.

LEARNING TO MEDITATE

Literally thousands of books have been written about meditation, which makes it seem intimidatingly complicated, and common misconceptions paint it as something mystical. Fortunately, it's neither of those things: meditation, or mindfulness as it is also called, is beautifully simple, and it's completely grounded in the real world around us.

You can meditate without any kind of outside guidance, but if you've never done it before then a little help will make it easier for you to build your confidence. The smartphone app Headspace is a popular starting point—I've used it myself many times—but there are plenty of other guided meditation resources out there.

The starting point for nearly all meditations is your breath. By focusing on the actions of inhaling and exhaling, we tune into our bodies and start to direct our thoughts to the moment that we are living in. Most of the time, you will close your eyes to remove external distractions. Think of these controlled, conscious breaths as the warm-up for the exercise that's to come. So all the meditations in this book open with simple breathing routines: you may find that you adapt them slightly according to what works best for you.

Once you are in tune with your breathing, the meditation will ask you to check in with your body, usually starting with the feet and working upwards. You will notice aches, itches, and physical tiredness, but you shouldn't judge or act on them; simply observe them, and move on to the next point in your body. This is a moment to acknowledge your body and feel grateful for all that it does for you. When your scan reaches your head, notice your emotional state. If you are angry, notice your anger—but don't succumb to it. If you are tired, or worried, or happy, or proud, notice the feeling, and name it, but don't judge it.

~~~~~~~~~~~~~~~~~~~~~~~~~~~~

Enjoy the moment!

~~~~~~~~~~~~~~~~~~~~~~~~~~~~

Now you've checked in with your body and your emotions, you can start on your surroundings and your place within them. In the bath, you'll notice how the water feels against your skin, how it supports your weight, and how it warms you. You'll register the fragrance of your essential oils—and every other smell in the room—and, again without judging, you'll hear the sounds around you, and the way the light falls. Name all these sights, sounds, smells, and sensations, then let them go.

If you suddenly realize that your mind has drifted away, simply note the thought, then gently redirect your attention back to where it was. Don't judge yourself when this happens— it's entirely natural, and it happens to everyone who meditates, every time they do so.

After a short time—most people start with meditations lasting about ten minutes—you will notice changes in how you feel. Your mind may be clearer, your muscles may be more relaxed, and your emotions may be calmer. As you meditate more often, you should find that this pleasant state becomes easier to reach—and lasts longer. You may want to do it for longer and longer periods, and you will probably find that you're more aware of your body, your emotions, and your surroundings. Enjoy the moment!

In order to really benefit from meditation, you need to do it often—ideally, daily. Every time you meditate, your brain reinforces the neural pathways in the white matter that help you think more clearly, stay calm, and feel happy. It's the same principle as with physical exercise: the more you do it, the more your muscles build, and the stronger you get. Another striking fact about meditation is that if you do it at the same time and in the same place every day, you will tend to benefit from it more. All the more reason to make it a fixture in your bathtime routine!

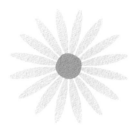

You'll notice that many of the meditations in this book start with the instruction to close your eyes. Obviously, when you do that you can't read the rest of the meditation! So prepare yourself before you start by reading through each meditation a couple of times.

This isn't an exam or a memory test, so don't worry about remembering it perfectly or peeking at the book to remind yourself. After a little practice you'll find that you can guide your own meditation and focus in a way that suits you.

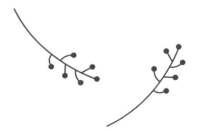

MUSIC TO DRIFT AWAY TO & MUSIC TO GET LOST IN

The only thing more relaxing than a warm, fragrant bath is a warm, fragrant bath with music. Most of us hear music every day—in stores, in our cars, on the radio, sometimes at work. But how often can we really pay attention to it and enjoy it to the full?

Giving you the time and space to relax into a piece, the bath is the perfect place to fall in love with something new, or listen closely to an old favorite and catch details that you haven't heard before. With your mind in its meditative, calm, focused state, you may find that it moves you more than ever.

There is plenty of evidence that our minds are hardwired to appreciate music. We have an inbuilt appreciation of rhythm, melody, and harmony, and

we find words that are sung have a greater emotional force than those that are spoken. Numerous academic studies have now proven that music is great for our mental health and well-being: our brains produce dopamine when we enjoy a song, which lifts our mood, and there's surprising evidence that patients recovering from operations need fewer painkilling drugs if they can listen to music (and fewer yet if they can choose the music themselves). It seems that music stimulates the production of natural opioids in the body, and also reduces levels of the stress hormone, cortisol. So that feeling of weightless euphoria that you experience when you put on your favorite song has real benefits.

Music doesn't just work on our minds, but on our bodies, too. We all know that upbeat music stimulates our cardiovascular system, making our heart pump more quickly, and causing us to breathe faster. Relaxing—lower-tempo—music has the opposite effect. We see a decrease in heart rate, we breathe more slowly, and our blood pressure drops. All of these effects are profoundly calming and relaxing, so if you're stressed, putting on a chilled-out tune is one of the best things you can do.

In order to avoid distraction, you should usually put on music after your meditation, visualization, or mindful practice. At the beginning of each section of bath treatments—Mind, Body, and Spirit—you'll find some general ideas about the kind of music that should make a good accompaniment to your spa, and I've also scattered a few personal choices throughout to spark ideas.

You should look on these specific recommendations as starting points for your own choices—suggestions, not prescriptions—after all, I can't tell you what you will enjoy! That said, I hope that you do give them a try and, maybe, discover something new. That profoundly relaxed, post-meditation state makes us particularly receptive to textures and tunes, and you may well find yourself enjoying a piece more than you ever have before.

PREPARING FOR YOUR HOME SPA

You shouldn't feel shy about setting aside a little time to look after yourself, and unwanted interruptions and distractions will stop you from enjoying your home spa to the full, so make sure they don't happen. If you have a single bathroom in your home, be sure to choose a time when it's not in high demand, such as late at night or early in the morning. Tell those you live with that you are occupying it and ask politely not to be disturbed. Let your family know that you are taking a half hour for yourself and will be back again afterwards with even more energy and love for them. And switch off your phone! You don't need to be alerted to *anything* right now.

Lock the door. Soften the lighting, light a candle, run the water, and if you want music, bring in a bluetooth speaker.

Don't race at the tub: the more relaxed you are when you get into the water, the more powerful its effects will be.

So before you get in, take a moment to stretch your arms, back, and legs, and roll your head gently to loosen any tight neck and shoulder muscles.

Make sure that your towel and robe are close at hand.

Close your eyes, breathe in deeply through your nose and out through your mouth, ten times. Test the water.

And step into your aromatic oasis.

THE
HOME SPA
RECIPES

Combining carefully selected essential oils with simple meditations and musical selections, each of these entries gives you everything you need for a restoring home spa treatment.

There are three sections—Mind, Body, and Spirit—and within each one you'll find a range of treatments, from the specific to the holistic. Pick one that you think you'll benefit from, spend a few minutes preparing for it—and enjoy!

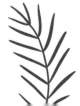

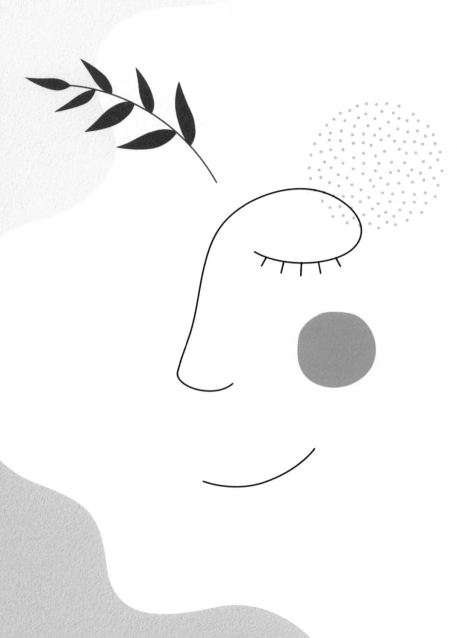

36

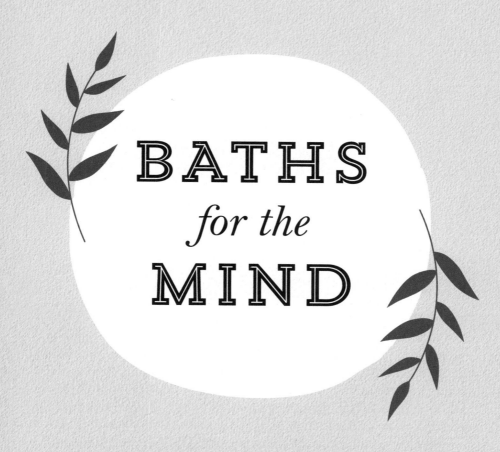

BATHS
for the
MIND

Most of us enjoy good mental health, most of the time, but that doesn't mean that we should neglect our minds and omit to give them a regular boost.

In this section, you'll combine aromatherapy, balneotherapy, meditation, and music to help your mind think more clearly, make good decisions, remain calm, and re-energize. And if you are feeling stressed, anxious, or troubled in any other way, a spa treatment can give you an invaluable lift.

CHOOSING MUSIC

I love all kinds of music—except for heavy
metal—but if I need to do some serious thinking,
I'll always turn to a classical piece.

Listening to the right kind of classical music will stimulate brain activity, letting you solve all kinds of mental problems—a phenomenon that some psychologists call "the Mozart Effect." We don't know exactly how it works, but it seems to be connected to the structures underpinning a classical piece, in which musical themes are repeated and varied in sophisticated ways. It's been found to help students study longer, remember more, and perform better in the exam hall.

But what is the right kind of classical music, and where do you begin if you don't usually listen to it?

Start with a piece without words or singing. Lyrics, and human voices, are particularly distracting when you're trying to focus. This means that you immediately rule out opera, choral music, and most religious music. I'd also avoid orchestral pieces and symphonies, which—especially if they're Beethoven's—often have dramatic contrasts between loud and quiet sections. This leaves small-scale pieces like quartets and trios, or solo performances. Finally, you don't want it to be too fast—something around 50–80 beats per minute is too slow to dance to, but gets your mind in the right place.

I love listening to solo piano works when I've got some particularly knotty brainwork to do. The intricate patterns of Bach's *Goldberg Variations* or *Partitas*, or Mozart's *Piano Sonatas* will make your mind click into a higher gear, and any of Chopin's piano works—try the *Mazurkas*—should have a similar effect. If you want something a little more emotional, but without the crashes and bangs of his symphonies, then try Beethoven's string quartets or piano trios. You will find numerous playlists online—search for "classical music for studying" and explore what's out there.

Many movie soundtracks, which are written to sink into the background as necessary, will have a similar effect, even if some are more electronic in feel. Some people swear by Hans Zimmer's work (try *Inception* or *Interstellar*), others by Trent Reznor (*The Social Network*, *Mank*), or Clint Mansell (*Pi*, *Moon*).

If you want to try something completely different, the sounds of nature, such as rain, waves on a beach, or the wind through trees, also enhance cognitive function and concentration. Even uninterrupted recordings work well, so search online for rainfall, ocean waves, and flowing streams.

FOR A MENTAL ENERGY BOOST

We are used to thinking of a relaxing bath, a soothing bath, or a sensual bath, but we don't often think of taking a bath to boost our brain power. But we should! Some of the best minds in history have had some of their greatest breakthroughs in the tub, all the way back to Archimedes shouting "Eureka!", and there's plenty of evidence that a spa session will boost your cranial computing power.

So if you're facing an exam, a test, or a particularly tricky professional challenge, then why not have a brain-training workout in the tub?

AROMAS & OILS

Numerous essential oils will help you think quicker and more clearly. Lemon brings balance, but also energy; Rosemary stimulates; and Bergamot unlocks concentration and creativity. So bring the bath to your preferred temperature, and add these oils as follows:

Lemon – 2 drops
Rosemary – 2 drops
Bergamot – 2 drops

MEDITATION

The focus and calm that mindfulness brings strengthen your mental muscles considerably, and it's great to see that schoolkids and students are now taught simple meditation techniques to help them learn. Anyone can benefit: studies show that meditation improves your cognitive processing ability.

This meditation brings tranquil strength and mental confidence.

Start by concentrating on your breaths. Give them your full attention—counting them may help you stay focused—inhaling slowly through your nose, then exhaling through your mouth. Notice how each breath differs from the one before, and register how deep, long, and steady each one is.

Now scan your body from the head down, noting all the sensations you find—discomforts, itches, aches, where you feel the water or the tub. Name every sensation, but don't judge anything. Feel yourself becoming more relaxed with every exhalation.

If your attention wanders at any point, gently return it to scanning and breathing.

Feel your head and face relaxing. As your breaths stay in this slow rhythm, imagine that each breath in brings in fresh air to clean out the cobwebs in your mind, and each breath out carries away some of the mental dust that's settled there. With each exhalation your body and mind will become more relaxed.

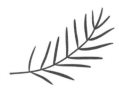

FOR A MENTAL DECLUTTER

Ever have the feeling that you've got too much to think about, too many things to remember? Every item on our mental to-do list demands energy and tires the brain so we don't have the strength to actually get stuff done. This spa treatment will help you declutter, regain focus, and prioritize.

You need to prepare yourself. Sit down with a pen and paper and make a list of everything that you've got on your mind— tasks that you need to do, people you need to contact, anything. Don't overcomplicate it: just write everything down, small and large, and take your time to try to avoid rushing and more tasks coming to the fore as soon as you're ready to relax. When that's done, tell yourself that the paper will remember everything for you— now, you can simply clear your mind and relax.

AROMAS & OILS

With your mind now free to let go, this heady mix of oils will help you find your center. Chamomile Roman brings peace; Lemongrass is calming and uplifting; Jasmine opens us so we can engage with the world again. Add them to the bath in these proportions just before stepping in.

Chamomile Roman – 3 drops
Lemongrass – 2 drops
Jasmine – 1 drop

MEDITATION

You should find that the act of writing down that list lightened your mental load considerably, and that the essential oils brought you to an open, peaceful frame of mind. Now a simple mindful meditation will help you center, and focus.

As ever, start by using your breath to get in tune with your body. Inhaling slowly through your mouth, then exhaling through your nose, count your breaths. Once you've got to ten, start again. Notice how each breath is always slightly different from the one before, and register how deep, long, and steady each one is.

Now scan your body from the head down, naming all the sensations you find—discomforts, itches, aches, where you feel the water or the tub. Notice and describe every sensation, but don't judge any of them. Feel your body relaxing with every exhalation.

If your attention wanders at any point, gently return it to scanning and breathing.

Picture each breath out carrying away distractions, and each breath in bringing focus and energy. If you find that you're thinking of an item on your to-do list, don't worry: simply note that you're thinking about it, and don't view it negatively. Then return to following your breaths, as they exchange tension for relaxation, confusion for clarity.

When you have followed your breaths to a point of deep relaxation, allow your mind to wander. Tell yourself that your list is full of opportunities to take a worthwhile action, and share positive energy with the world.

A BURNOUT RECOVERY BATH

The brain can only take so much hard studying or heavy, intellectual work. If you're burying yourself in a difficult project, concentrating hard every day, it's going to run out of energy at some point and take you to the nasty point that we call burnout. Time to recharge your batteries.

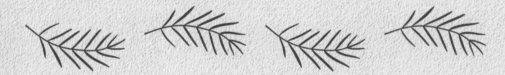

AROMAS & OILS

In this mixture, Rosemary and Basil bring stimulating qualities, and Lemon, as always, restores balance. Run your bath, check that the temperature is right, then add the oils as follows:

Rosemary – 2 drops
Basil – 2 drops
Lemon – 3 drops

MEDITATION

Burnout is a horrible combination of tiredness and nervous energy. Our reserves are depleted, and our body and brain make up for this by running on adrenaline—which is a useful strategy in the very short term, but it becomes damaging if it lasts for too long.

The best thing you can do is to center yourself, conserving positive energy and channeling it around your body. Whatever challenges you face will be easier to deal with if you are calm and refreshed, so this mindful meditation is all about reducing tension and recharging your batteries.

Relax into the bath and feel the essential oils starting to do their work.

Then give all your limbs a shake, throwing off the nervous energy and making them as loose as possible. Start to focus on your breathing: inhale slowly and deeply through your mouth, then exhale through your nose. Count your breaths and notice how they become slower, steadier, and more even. With each breath in, feel the air's positive energy; with each breath out, notice your joints, limbs, and chest relaxing.

When you have counted to ten, return to zero and go again. Carry on until you can feel your heart rate dropping and a relaxed calm spreading through your whole body. Now scan your body from feet to head, noticing how each part feels as you move your attention slowly up. Notice and name any aches or other sensations, but don't judge them. If you notice your train of thought going off-track, don't worry: just redirect your attention to where it should be.

When you've checked in with your whole body, work back through it, tensing your muscles as you breathe in and relaxing them as you breathe out. Tense and relax your neck and shoulders this way first, for a few breaths, and then move down your arms to your fingers, then down your torso and legs to your toes. With each exhalation, picture tension leaving your muscles and calm flooding in to replace it.

SOUNDS

For burnout you want something that's emotional but not excitable. Why not let Billie Holiday pull you into her world with her unique voice? She recorded hundreds of deeply moving numbers—and she sang about getting over the bad times better than anyone.

45

FOR CONFIDENCE & ASSERTIVENESS

Confidence is one of the most important, empowering, and attractive attributes; we need it every day, but on some occasions—first dates, presentations, and job interviews, for instance—it becomes particularly important. Those are the times when you need to believe in yourself and know that when you speak, you deserve to be heard.

AROMAS & OILS

This heady mixture will fill you with faith in yourself and your abilities. The two woody oils will empower you and make you feel strong, while Jasmine has been called "the shy person's best friend" for its confidence-inspiring properties. So take a few deep breaths, stretch your arms and back up as far as they will go, then add these oils to your bath in these proportions—and step in.

Cedarwood – 3 drops
Rosemary – 2 drops
Jasmine – 2 drops

MEDITATION

This meditation uses the power of visualization to give you that additional boost. By picturing yourself projecting confidence and saying what you need to say, you can make it happen. As always, though, it starts with controlled breathing.

Sink into the bath, letting the essential oils work their magic.

Stretch out each of your limbs, shaking out any restlessness or tension.

Then focus on the breaths you take: inhaling slowly and deeply through your mouth, before exhaling through your nose. Count your breaths and notice how they become slower, steadier, and more even.

When your body is relaxed, start to repeat the word "confidence" to yourself with each breath in. Say it as a mantra, feeling confidence fill your whole body, from the lungs outwards. If your attention should wander, don't worry, just return to your mantra.

When you can feel the idea of confidence with every part of your body, visualize yourself expressing it. Picture what you have to do tomorrow: see yourself with other people, going through the normal routine, standing tall, and with your eyes shining. Picture yourself speaking clearly and being heard. Picture yourself making eye contact, smiling, laughing. Picture yourself as you wish to be seen by others.

Return to the "confidence" mantra, and feel yourself becoming more and more self-assured.

FOR WILLPOWER & DETERMINATION

The noted wellness author Oliver Burkeman has written that "the ability to tolerate minor discomfort is a superpower," and he's right. How often do we let small amounts of boredom, worry, or irritation stop us from getting things done? How often do we procrastinate, even knowing that it will cause us problems? How often do you find yourself wishing you had the willpower just to get on with things, and to make progress?

AROMAS & OILS

This woody blend will boost your mental strength, giving you the resolve you need to focus and finish the job—whatever that happens to be. Cedarwood warms you psychologically as well as physically, and brings a calming strength that will help you concentrate.

Meanwhile, Cypress helps you through transitions, and this session is all about transition, change, and movement. Drop the oils into the bath as follows:

Cypress – 4 drops
Cedarwood – 4 drops

MEDITATION

Burkeman suggests that you can increase your capacity for discomfort—in effect, gaining willpower to take on difficult or boring tasks—in the same way as you train at the gym. With practice, when you find feelings of irritability, anxiety, or boredom rising, you can watch them mindfully, letting them arise and fade, while carrying on with the task anyway. "The rewards come so quickly, in terms of what you'll accomplish," he says, "that it soon becomes the more appealing way to live."

So this "emotion-surfing" mindfulness exercise isn't just for your spa. Instead, it's an exercise that you can carry out whenever you feel yourself losing the willpower that you need to complete an unpleasant task. It's based on a routine by Bernadette Dijkhuizen-Keogh.

Remember that no emotion is permanent. Boredom, frustration, and irritation all come and go: the trick is to acknowledge these feelings and name them. So regularly tune in to how you feel, and note those feelings: "I feel frustrated," or "I'm feeling relaxed," or "I feel disappointed."

Don't judge these feelings. They are what they are, neither good nor bad, just natural. Accept that they are how you feel right now, and give yourself permission to feel that way.

Try to place that emotion in your body. Do you feel it in your chest, in your jaw, in your head, in your hands? Tell yourself where it is, and how it affects your body.

Then ask yourself, "I wonder where this emotion comes from?" If it's from a frustrating situation, or a task you need to take on, then connect the two, but don't make any judgments. Always be kind to yourself. Observe the connection between thoughts and feelings, but don't beat yourself up about them.

In short: once you have noticed the feelings that are stopping you from getting stuff done, just name them, examine them, locate them in your body, and ask yourself calmly where they come from—all without judgment. This is "emotion surfing," and you'll find that it will remove all kinds of obstacles from your life!

TO FIND THE ANSWER

You need to face big decisions with a clear head. You may be considering a house move, a new job, ending or starting a relationship: whatever it is, you want your body relaxed and your mind clear. This spa treatment will bring clarity, helping you to strip away what's unnecessary and focus on the essentials, and the meditation will make you frame the question in a new, constructive way.

AROMAS & OILS

Basil, Cardamom, Rosemary, and Lemon are your essential oils for this mission. Cardamom lifts the spirits and inspires courage; Lemon brings balance and clarity; Rosemary helps when you need to analyze a problem; and Basil perks up the brain, giving you an uplifting boost. Together they will help you find the best way forwards. Gather the bottles, run the bath, and when it's ready, add the oils as follows:

Basil – 3 drops
Cardamom – 3 drops
Rosemary – 2 drops
Lemon – 2 drops

MEDITATION

Step into the bath, have a stretch and shake, then turn your mind to the problem you need to solve.

It can seem impossible to balance life's conflicting priorities, and decisions are difficult when we try to satisfy the demands of our career, our reputation, our relationships, our physical comfort, and our commitments to others. Often, when we ask "What's best for me?" or "What will make me happy?", we're actually asking the wrong question. In his book *What Matters Most*, the psychoanalyst and author James Hollis came up with an ingenious way to reframe these questions:

"Ask yourself of every dilemma, every choice, every relationship, every commitment, or every failure to commit: Does this choice diminish me, or enlarge me?"

His belief is that if you choose to enlarge yourself, rather than close down your horizons, you will live a more meaningful—and therefore happier—life. This meditation frames that question for you.

As always, use controlled breathing exercises to center yourself and remove distractions from your mind.

When your body is relaxed and you are breathing steadily and calmly, turn your mind to the question that you need to answer. Notice how you feel about the different alternatives. Are you excited? Worried? Unconfident? Is it about money? Are you concerned at the effect your decision will have on others? Name these emotions, without judging them: ask yourself where they come from, but don't be hard on yourself.

When you've looked at all of the emotions around your dilemma or decision, ask yourself the question in a different way: "Does this choice diminish me or enlarge me?" Consider how each option will encourage you to grow as a person. Which will challenge you positively? Which will bring rewards in the long term, not just right now?

Carry on breathing steadily until insights arrive...

TO COOL DOWN & CALM DOWN

There's another bath for physical heat on page 88, but this one here is all about reducing the emotional temperature—if you're riled about something, or fear that you may say something that you'll come to regret.

AROMAS & OILS

Lemon is, as ever, appropriate because it restores balance and brings you back towards a natural equilibrium. Chamomile Roman is deeply calming, and Marjoram reduces stress and makes you feel secure. When the bath is full, add the oils in the following proportions, and slip in calmly.

Lemon – 2 drops
Chamomile Roman – 3 drops
Marjoram – 3 drops

MEDITATION

It may take you a little while to get your head in the right place to meditate, and that's fine. Simply relax in the bath, close your eyes, maybe listen to a little music, and take your mind off whatever it is that has riled you.

Then breathe calmly and deeply, counting each breath, until you are more relaxed. With each breath in, feel yourself cooling down; with each breath out, expel hot, angry air. Pay close attention to your breaths, noting how each is different from the one before. If you notice your attention

wandering away, gently return it to your breath.

When you're completely relaxed, have a close look at what it is that's bothered you. Note the emotions that it arouses, but don't judge them—even if the emotions are impatience, anger, and frustration! Instead, name the emotions, and lift them up—like a rock on the seashore—to see what lies beneath. Note your own sensitivities and vulnerabilities, but, again, don't judge or reprimand yourself.

If it's a person who's close to you that you're angry with, then try a gratitude exercise: identify five ways in which this person enriches your life. They may challenge you, but they may also help you, make you laugh, or expose you to new things. Remind yourself how grateful you are to the universe for bringing that person into your life.

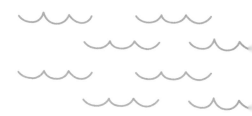

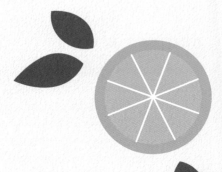

TO PREPARE
FOR A BIG
DAY AHEAD

It might be a job interview, it might be an exam, it might be your wedding day: from time to time, life throws up moments when you really have to be on top of your game. This spa treatment and visualization will help you clear your head, refresh your batteries, and envision a complete success.

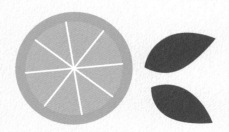

AROMAS & OILS

The oils in this mixture will boost your powers of concentration and focus—helping you visualize effectively—and will strengthen your faith and emotional resolve. Lemon brings clarity, as does Rosemary, which also helps your visual imagination. Sandalwood will give you the emotional confidence to imagine a perfect outcome to the challenge you face.

So fill a tub, take a few deep breaths, then add these powerful oils and get ready for a bracing, fortifying, spa treatment.

Lemon – 3 drops
Sandalwood – 3 drops
Rosemary – 2 drops

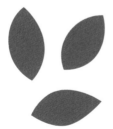

MEDITATION

You're not just daydreaming, there's now plenty of scientific and psychological research to demonstrate that visualizing a successful outcome to a challenge is one of the best ways to help you accomplish it. Leading athletes and sportspeople have known this for years: one study found that basketball players who just pictured themselves making successful free throws improved as quickly as those who actually practiced with the ball!

So time spent visualizing—or mentally rehearsing—is definitely not time wasted. →

SOUNDS

This is an opportunity to take full advantage of classical music's brain-boosting qualities. Try Beethoven's *Diabelli Variations*, an intricate series of short piano pieces, or Erik Satie's playful solo works.

You need to create sensory and emotional impressions for this to really work, so imagine how the parts of your visualization sound, look, feel, and smell, and note the emotions that you feel during it, too.

If you just picture yourself in the "third person"—as if you were a character in a movie—it won't work. You need to visualize everything from your own point of view, as seen through your own eyes, in the "first person." You have to picture yourself there— in the exam room, in the interview room, on the basketball court— seeing what you'll see, hearing the noises that you'll hear, wearing the clothes that you'll wear, and so on. Feel the pencil, resumé, ring, or ball in your hand.

As the basketball coach Joe Haefner puts it: "As you shoot, you should FEEL the ball roll off your fingers. You should SEE the ball traveling through the air with perfect backspin. You should SEE your hands out in front of you with the perfect follow-through. You should SEE your hands out in front of you holding the follow-through as you HEAR and SEE the ball swish through the net."

So picture every part of the scene that you're preparing for, and every move that you'll make, all the way through to a completely successful result. Concentrate on the details, the emotions, and your own point of view.

Then run through it again, and again. Repetition works!

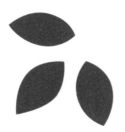

Concentrate on the details,
the emotions, and your own
point of view

FOR CONCENTRATION & ANALYSIS

We sometimes forget how much fun hard work can be! Writing a term paper can be an absorbing, enthralling experience—the hours will fly by, if you are confident with what you're doing. The same applies to compiling a business's accounts, preparing a presentation, or even writing a company report. Tricky yet achievable tasks are the most satisfying that we have— if you are able to concentrate on them.

This spa treatment and visualization will give the frontal lobes of your brain a timely boost, so you can power through the task at hand with concentrated attention. It may make sense to do it in the morning—or the afternoon, come to that—and that's absolutely fine!

AROMAS & OILS

To prepare for your brain work, you need Lemon, supplemented with Basil and Rosemary. Step into the tub and take a few moments simply to inhale and appreciate.

Lemon – 3 drops
Basil – 3 drops
Rosemary – 2 drops

58

EXERCISES

In just three steps, these simple visualization exercises will train your brain to focus intently and creatively. Use them as a warm-up for the task at hand, and practice them regularly to build up your powers of concentration and focus. These are deliberately sequenced to turn your attention from the outside world—and the past—to your own capabilities, and the future.

Rerun Your Day

Close your eyes, and review in your mind the day's events so far. As if you've been living a movie, replay everything that's happened and everything you've done, from the second you woke up to this very moment. Recall as much detail as you can: places, faces, colors, sounds, and smells.

Clone the Shampoo Bottle

Now place a simple object—it can be anything near at hand; it doesn't necessarily have to be a bottle of shampoo—on the side of the bath where you can focus on it. Observe it closely for two minutes, studying all its details: texture, shape, color, material, pattern. Keep your mind on it and when you notice your mind wandering, return your focus to the object. After two minutes, close your eyes and replicate the bottle in your mind's eye. Keep the mental picture detailed, clear, and stable for at least a minute. It may fade or change as you do so, but don't worry, just keep focused.

Visualizing Handwriting

For the third exercise, close your eyes and picture a blank sheet of paper and a fountain pen in your hand. Slowly write your name, letter by letter, in blue letters, watching the letters run across the page. You'll probably find it difficult to hold all of the letters that you've written in mind, but keep practicing until your name is complete. Your focus and powers of visualization will improve over time.

Remember that your brain burns up a *lot* of energy. While you're working, keep your blood sugar levels steady with a banana or similar snack—something healthy that releases energy over time, not processed fats and sugars.

TO STOP PROCRASTINATION

It's horrible to realize that you've procrastinated yourself into unhappiness. One of our most stressful emotions must be that underlying worry that we're forgetting things, that we're not getting them done in good time, that we're letting others down, or not making the most of life's opportunities. The good news is that it's relatively easy to shake off the bad mental habits that lead you into this kind of situation, and this treatment, designed to be regularly repeated, uses a powerful combination of essential oils and visualizations to help you adopt good habits. Try it, and bring a reassuring order to your life!

Before you start the bath, make a list of everything that you've got to do, including everything that you've procrastinated about. (Perhaps try using a pencil or crayon, to avoid smudging later.) It might include shopping, bills that you need to pay, dates that you need to arrange, work tasks—everything that's on your mind right now. Take your time and take care that your list is complete, and be sure to include those jobs that you've been putting off for a while. It may be quite a long list! (The last time I did this exercise, my own was twenty-six entries long.)

Now decide on the one or two big tasks that you want to get done the most, which you can get done in the next day—if you stop putting them off! Make a mark next to each of them on the list. Then pick three or four smaller tasks that you know you can also fit in. Place your list where you can see it from the tub—you'll be referring to the items on it.

AROMAS & OILS

To the bath, add the following oils: Lemon for clarity and purpose, Eucalyptus for liberation, and Rosemary for alertness and stimulation. Then don't delay: stepping into the water is the first step towards getting everything done!

Lemon – 2 drops
Rosemary – 2 drops
Eucalyptus – 2 drops

MEDITATION

Once you are thoroughly relaxed, and you can feel the essential oils doing their work, carry out this visualization exercise.

Breathe calmly and deeply, counting each breath, until you are relaxed. With each breath in, feel yourself becoming calmer: with each breath out, expel confusion. As ever, pay close attention to your breaths, noting how each is different from the one before: if you notice your attention wandering, gently return it to your breathing.

Once you have counted twenty or thirty breaths in this way, turn your attention to the list. Look at the first item on it: picture yourself completing it and doing a great job. Imagine the scene in detail: where are you? What actions are you making? How will you feel when this task is done? How long will it take? Create a clear image of success in your mind. Repeat the sequence at least once. Picture yourself crossing the item off the list.

Now move on to the next item, and repeat the process, vividly imagining yourself successfully completing the next job and crossing it off the list.

The next day, don't delay: go straight into the first job on the list. Carry it out as you visualized it yesterday. When you've struck all of the targeted jobs off your list, identify the next batch that you should do, and tonight repeat the process.

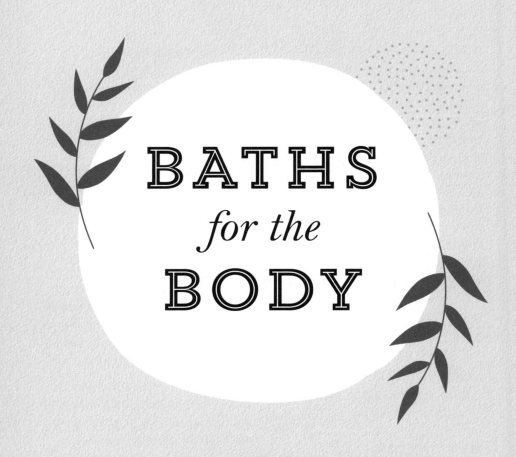

BATHS
for the
BODY

We all know that soaking in a hot bath is a terrific way to relax our muscles and joints, but the benefits don't end there. Many essential oils have quite specific effects on the other organs of our body, including the digestive, circulation, and respiratory systems. Combine that with a meditation session that itself reduces damaging stress hormones like cortisone, and you'll never feel better.

CHOOSING MUSIC

There's good medical evidence that listening to music helps the body heal from illnesses, injuries, or operations. The psychological boost that it gives us—lowering stress, making us happier, taking our mind off pain—makes a massive difference to how quickly our body recovers, and it seems to be thanks to the effect that music has on our hormones. Music triggers the release of oxytocin, the "love hormone" that reduces the levels of pain we experience. At the same time, it reduces levels of cortisol, the stress hormone that makes inflammation worse, and increases levels of dopamine and serotonin, the hormones of happiness that help your body recover from exertion.

So what kind of music works best? In brief: music that you like! If your aim with this bath treatment is to soothe an ache or get over a strenuous workout, then just put on a playlist of your favorites, and relax with some familiar pleasures.

FOR A GOOD NIGHT'S SLEEP

Insomnia can be the most frustrating of all ailments. There is nothing worse than lying awake in the small hours, desperate to sleep, and fearful that sleep will not come. Thankfully, it is possible to build an evening routine that will help—and this bath treatment can be a part of it.

Firstly, you should check that you're not doing anything that is already significantly affecting your sleeping patterns. Cut down on caffeinated drinks (not just coffee and tea: many soft drinks have high levels of caffeine, too) and avoid bright screens for a couple of hours before bedtime.

Take a bath an hour or so before bed, and afterwards read a book, or listen to an audiobook or podcast. This mixture of oils will help you, but be careful not to apply too much, as it may be overly stimulating! For the same reason, run this bath warm, but not too hot—you want to avoid cardiovascular stimulation at this time of day. When you dip your hand in to test it, there shouldn't be any kind of tingle, just a feeling of comfort. Finally, this spa treatment definitely works best by candlelight. You don't need a scented candle: it's the muted, calming quality of the light that's important.

> Dim the lights throughout your home for a couple of hours before bedtime.

AROMAS & OILS

When the tub's ready, and the light is low, add the oils in the following proportions, and slip in gently.

Clary Sage – 2 drops
Vetiver – 1 drop
Lavender – 1 drop

MEDITATION

We know that mindfulness improves our night's rest by increasing levels of melatonin, a natural hormone which makes us sleepy, and at the same time reducing levels of the stress hormone cortisol. It will also reduce anxiety and other negative thoughts that can buzz around our heads and keep us awake. This meditation is focused on the body, and the night drawing in around you. →

Close your eyes. Begin as usual by noticing and guiding your breaths: inhale through your nose for a second, hold your breath for two seconds, then exhale for five seconds or longer. Repeat this twenty times, counting as you inhale. Notice the flow of air through your mouth and nose, the movements of your chest as you inhale and exhale, and the fact that every breath is unique.

With your eyes closed, carry on breathing steadily and meditatively, and work your way up your body, noticing how your feet and legs feel after carrying you through the day. Work up through the trunk of your body, through your shoulders and arms to your fingertips and the top of your head. Notice how your body feels, but don't judge. Then start to tense up and relax the muscles in each area, from your feet up. Hold the tension for a couple of breaths each time.

Now notice the sounds of evening falling, and the world becoming quieter around you. If your bathroom has a window, watch the sky darkening: if it doesn't, notice the shadows cast by your flickering candle.

Close your eyes again and repeat the opening breathing exercise.

Notice the sounds of evening falling, and the world becoming quieter around you

MUSIC FOR GOOD SLEEP

Way back in 1741, the composer Bach was commissioned to create a set of variations for an insomniac Russian aristocrat, Count Kaiserling. The plan was that Kaiserling's clavier player, one Johann Gottlieb Goldberg, would perform them each night outside his chamber, helping his master to drop off. And they worked—so effectively, that Kaiserling listened to them at bedtime regularly for years. Well… that's the story, anyway. Sadly, there's probably no truth to it. But Bach's *Goldberg Variations* are undeniably a wonderful way to wind down at the end of the day. There are many recorded versions online, including remarkable solo piano performances from Angela Hewitt and Glenn Gould.

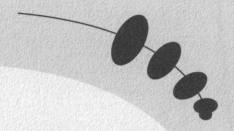

TO RECOVER AFTER EXERTION

There's something wonderful about sliding exhausted muscles into a warm bath. Whether you've been hard at work, or you've pushed your body at the gym, nothing's better than letting the water take your weight. With a selection of robust, powerful oils, this bath will boost your recovery so that you come back even stronger, and ready to go the next day.

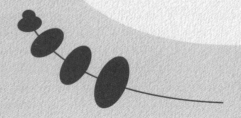

AROMAS & OILS

Lavender helps tissue to recover from exertion; Eucalyptus is an antiinflammatory; and Ginger is good for the ligaments and joints. Together they create a heady aroma, so once you've dropped the oils in, inhale deeply through your nose.

Ginger – 1 drop
Eucalyptus – 2 drops
Lavender – 2 drops

You can add bath salts (or Epsom Salts) to this bath without changing how the essential oils work. They have their own powerful effects on muscle aches and pains and will make this treatment even more effective.

MEDITATION

Identifying aches and pains will make them less powerful, and this meditation combines mindful observation with some gentle stretches.

Begin as usual by controlling and observing your breaths. Inhale through your nose for a second: hold your breath for a couple of seconds, then breathe out over five seconds or more. Count each time and repeat ten times.

Now it's time to acknowledge your body's hard work. Begin with the soles of the feet: notice how they feel, and how the water laps around your toes. Stretch your feet, pointing your toes a few times so that you can feel the muscles tensing. Notice any aches and pains, but don't judge them.

Then slowly work your way up your body, and check in with your legs, your joints, your trunk, and so on; tense, then relax the muscles in each area, and notice how they feel. When you arrive at the shoulders, roll them backwards and forwards, noticing how the muscles in your back, shoulders, and arms work together. Stretch your arms out forwards a few times, extending your fingers: clench then unclench your fists. Lift one leg to your chest, and hug it tightly with both arms, breathing steadily all the time. Repeat with your other leg.

Finally, close your eyes and feel the muscles in your neck as you slowly push your head forwards, then back. Let the bath take your weight and notice the sensation of aches steadily fading away.

A FRIDAY NIGHT WIND-DOWN

The bridge between an exhausting time at work and a precious couple of days to ourselves, Friday night is one of the most important moments in the week. Make the most of it with this revitalizing treatment; it makes the cares of the week recede, and energizes you to make the most of your own time.

AROMAS & OILS

This uses a combination of essential oils to create a healing, yet stimulating atmosphere. Geranium is a calming, comforting aroma that feels a lot like coming home; Lavender, one of the most powerful of all the essential oils, reduces jitteriness and worry; and Neroli (Orange Blossom) will move you forwards with feelings of calm and regeneration.

Run the bath and add the oils, as follows, before you climb in.

Lavender – 2 drops
Geranium – 1 drop
Neroli – 1 drop

Breathe slowly and deeply through your nose for at least ten minutes.

Of course, for many people, the "Friday night moment" doesn't actually happen on a Friday night! But don't worry, if you work weekends, or irregularly, you can run this bath treatment anytime you've finished work and have a little time to yourself coming up.

CANDLELIGHT

The perfect complement to this mix is a candle dispersing another layer of Neroli. This is a common aroma in scented candles, so it will be easy to obtain one if you want: alternatively, make your own by letting a wide unscented candle burn until it has formed a puddle of melted wax (you should light it 20 minutes or so before your bath time). When you add the essential oils to your bath, also add a couple of drops to the melted wax, away from the flame (you want the oil to evaporate, not burn).

MEDITATION

Once you've been in the bath for a few minutes, inhaling the essential oils and starting to decompress, turn to this meditation.

Begin with a simple breathing exercise: breathe in through your nose for a second: hold your breath for two seconds, then breathe out over five seconds or more. Repeat this ten times, noticing the flow of air through your mouth and nose, the movements of your chest as you inhale and exhale, and the fact →

that every breath is slightly different from the one before.

Now it's time to acknowledge the body that has carried you through a week of hard graft: commuting, working, helping others, and earning your living. Start with the feet: notice how they feel, how they are relaxing now that you've taken your weight off them, and how the water moves around them and between your toes. Notice any aches and pains, but don't judge them, or feel bad about them. Stretch your feet, pointing your toes a few times so that you are conscious of how the muscles control them and are connected to your joints. Thank your feet for the work they've done for you this week, and acknowledge how important they will be for the weekend ahead.

SOUNDS

This is a time to really indulge yourself with pure pleasure: lush, tuneful, upbeat music—try disco or dance music, or party tunes!

Promise them a gentle stroll, or a walk on grass, a jog, or a swim; any form of exercise that is just about feeling positive and looking after yourself.

Then work your way up your body, checking in with your legs, your joints, your abdomen, and so on: tense, then relax the muscles in each area, and notice how they feel. Thank each part in turn for how it has supported you through the week, and how it will help you get the most from the free time ahead.

When you come to the shoulders, roll them backwards and forwards a few times, noticing how the muscles in your back, shoulders, and arms work together. Stretch your arms out forwards a few times, extending your fingers as far as they will go: clench and unclench your fists, thinking about how the joints in your fingers work together. Acknowledge your hands and thank them for all they have done for you this week, and let them simply float freely in the warm water: notice how buoyant they feel.

Finally, close your eyes and concentrate on the muscles in your neck. Feel the water around it; let the bath take the weight of your head, if you like. Use your senses: listen actively to the music, to how the rhythms, melodies, and harmonies develop. Notice the aromas in the room, the way the steam rises, and the play of candlelight and shadow. Breathe steadily, and you will feel your body move away from the stresses of the week and towards the pleasures of the weekend.

Breathe steadily, and you will feel your body move away from the stresses of the week and towards the pleasures of the weekend

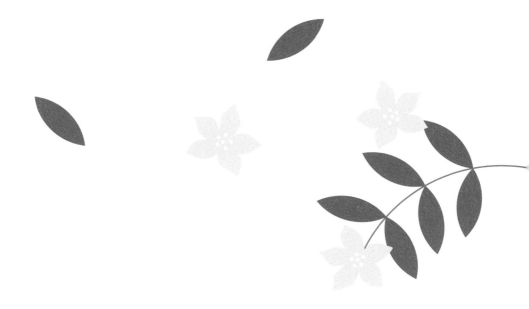

FOR MUSCLE ACHES & PAINS

A hot bath on its own will do aching muscles the world of good, but if you combine some healing oils and the gentle stretches of a mindfulness scan, the benefits can be amazing.

AROMAS & OILS

This simple spa treatment combines Rosemary, which is known for its powerful effect on our muscles, with Lemongrass, which is equally good for our "soft" connective tissues like ligaments and tendons. Add the oils to your bath as below, and have a good stretch of your arms and back before you step into the water.

Rosemary – 4 drops
Lemongrass – 4 drops

MEDITATION

This simple, mindful stretching routine will help you loosen up even more, and squeeze painful lactic acids out of your muscles.

Close your eyes. Breathing deeply and slowly, in through your nose, then out through your mouth, feel the oxygen bringing a clean energy into your body. As you exhale, feel your relaxation deepen and deepen. Notice how the water warms your muscles and takes the weight off your joints.

Scan up your body from your toes to the top of your head, noticing any aches and pains, and naming them without judging them. If you can, name the cause of each ache. Notice your joints: the ankles, knees, hips, and shoulders in particular. If they are tight, focus on them, and soften them with each exhalation.

Stretch the muscles of one leg, pointing your toes so it is absolutely extended, and hold it tense for two breaths. (You may need to lift it out of the bath.) Breathe steadily in through your nose, out through your mouth as you do. Repeat with the second leg, and notice how the muscles feel after each stretch. Now continue to your arms, stretching, clenching your fists, then relaxing them after a couple of breaths. Gently direct your head to left and then right, stretching your neck without straining it, before rolling your head gently around to loosen your shoulder and neck.

Now scan your body again, noticing how the stretches have changed how it feels. Then notice your whole body, present in this moment. Return your attention to your breathing until you are ready to open your eyes again.

FOR TENSION & TIGHTNESS

Stress and anxiety can bury themselves deep in our bodies, causing our muscles to hold themselves tightly and eventually stiffen up with pain.

If you have tense muscles, stretch them out gently for a few minutes before you climb into the bath: hold your arms outwards and rotate them to loosen your shoulders and chest. Rotate your torso from side to side, then bend to touch your toes a few times—don't worry if you can't reach them.

AROMAS & OILS

Ginger, Chamomile, and Nutmeg are all good oils for muscular and soft-tissue aches. Marjoram, in small quantities, reduces tension too. Add your oils to the bath in the proportions below, then take a deep breath and slip into the welcoming water.

Ginger – 1 drop
Chamomile – 3 drops
Nutmeg – 2 drops
Marjoram – 1 drop

This sweet, heady blend will work particularly well in a bath crystal mixture (see page 20).

MEDITATION

A good way to reduce the severity of the pain you experience is to separate the objective sensory aspect and the subjective judgment that we make of them. We can think of a twisted knee as being "horribly painful" or we can notice the pain and observe— neutrally—that our body is telling us that something isn't right in the knee and that it needs to heal. This mindful body scan will help you to step back from your pain in this way, and put it in the context of your whole body.

Close your eyes. Take a few deep breaths in through your nose, out through your mouth. As you inhale, feel the oxygen bringing life to the body, and as you exhale, feel your relaxation deepen and deepen. Notice the water on your skin, your feet touching the end of the tub. The water warms you, carries your weight, presses lightly onto your body.

Notice your legs, their heaviness, and lightness. Name any aches and pains that you come across in your scan, but don't judge them. Notice your torso, how it swells and contracts with your breaths, and pay attention to your stomach. If it is tense or tight, let it soften. Breathe steadily in through your nose, out through your mouth, all the time.

Notice the joints: ankles, knees, hips, shoulders, elbows, wrists. Are they tense or tight? See if they will soften. Notice any pain without judging it. In this way, scan your whole body until you are completely aware of every sensation in it. Then notice your whole body, present in this moment. Carry on breathing steadily until you are ready to open your eyes again.

TO GET OVER ILLNESS

Too often our impatience pushes us to rush our recovery from infections, illness, or disease, and we underestimate exactly how much energy the body needs to put into the recovery process. We hurry back to our feet, or back to work, and as a result put back our recovery or end up ill again. This bath combines restorative essential oils with a mindful body scan that will tune you in to how your body really is— not how you want it to be. Use it to keep yourself on a steady path of recovery and recuperation.

AROMAS & OILS

This is a good all-purpose mixture which will boost your mental and physical health alike. The Chamomile, in particular, will lift your spirits; Coriander will also cheer you, and boost your appetite; Geranium is cheering and positive; and Lavender is a good all-round tonic. Add the oils in the below proportions, and lower yourself gently into the supportive, nurturing water.

Coriander – 2 drops
Chamomile – 2 drops
Geranium – 2 drops
Lavender – 2 drops

MEDITATION

This simple body scan will help you to tune in with your body as it recovers from illness.

Close your eyes. Take a few deep breaths in through your nose, then out through your mouth. As you inhale, feel the oxygen bringing life to the body, and as you exhale, feel your relaxation deepen. Notice the water on your body, and the soles of your feet on the end of the tub.

The water warms you, carries your weight, presses lightly on your skin.

Scan up your body, noticing any itches, aches, and pains, and naming them without judging them. Notice the weight of your legs and feel them relax as you exhale, and pay attention to your stomach. Notice how your chest swells and contracts with your breaths. If it is tense or tight, let it soften. Breathe steadily in through your nose, out through your mouth, all the time. Feel the air passing through the airways of your nose, mouth, throat, and chest, and fill your lungs as deeply as you can. Notice any parts that bear the signs of your illness. Observe any aches or pains and name them, knowing that they will diminish as you recover. Notice the joints that have been underused while you've been unwell: ankles, knees, hips, shoulders, elbows, wrists. Are they tense or tight? See if they will soften.

In this way, scan your whole body. Then notice your whole body, present in this moment, on a journey back to health. Breathe steadily until you are ready to open your eyes.

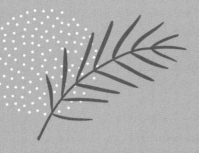

AN IMMUNITY BOOSTER

We've all become much more aware of how infections pass from person to person in recent years. There's plenty you can do to make yourself more disease-resistant, without isolating yourself: moderate exercise (but not heavy training; champion athletes in peak condition are notoriously susceptible to coughs and colds), fresh air, and plenty of fruit and vegetables.

But if you know that you're going to be mixing with hundreds of people, and there are coughs, colds, and flu around, you can take this bath treatment, too, which will give your immune system a short-term boost.

AROMAS & OILS

Four oils work together in this treatment. Tea Tree brings antiviral, antibacterial and antifungal qualities; Geranium and Lavender are both antiseptic; and Rosemary gives the body a handy little pick-me-up. Add the oils drop by drop as directed below, then get into the water and inhale deeply.

> *Tea Tree* – 2 drops
> *Geranium* – 1 drop
> *Lavender* – 1 drop
> *Rosemary* – 2 drops

Remember that, like all aromatherapy treatments, the effects of this mixture aren't long-lasting, so you should use it daily, for as long as you know that your immune system will be exposed to higher than usual numbers of people. You can mix the oils in advance, or make your own candle or diffuser. Happily, it smells wonderful too!

MEDITATION

There's now plenty of medical research that proves beyond doubt what many regular meditators already suspected: mindfulness boosts your immune system. There seem to be three main ways in which this works.

Firstly, your immune system is highly susceptible to stress, and anything that reduces stress therefore helps it. Mindfulness reduces inflammation by helping us to think positively, not ruminate or dwell on negative subjects. Another mechanism, connecting our minds directly to our immune system, involves CD-4 blood cells, which carry messages for our white blood cells, and telomerase, a protein that protects our chromosomes and therefore slows aging and cancer. Finally, mindfulness can boost immunity in the gut microbiota—the trillions of tiny organisms that break down and digest our food for us, and protect us from a host of nasty infections. Regular practice will help your gut microbiota stay strong and well balanced. →

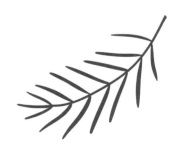

So regular mindfulness will really help you fight off infections and disease. Performing a simple body scan meditation every day, like the one on page 77, is a great place to begin.

Start by focusing on your breaths. Give them all your attention—counting them may help you stay focused—inhaling deeply through your nose, then exhaling slowly through your mouth. Aim to fill your torso with each breath, starting at the diaphragm and drawing air in until your chest is completely expanded. Notice how each breath differs from the one that preceded it, and register how deep, long, and steady each one is.

Now scan your body from the feet up, noting all the feelings and sensations you find—discomforts, itches, aches, where you feel the water or the tub. Name every sensation, but don't judge anything or react to them. Feel yourself becoming more relaxed with every exhalation as your muscles and joints loosen.

If your attention wanders, gently return it to scanning and breathing.

Feel your head and face relaxing. As your breaths stay in this slow rhythm, tell yourself that each breath in brings with it strength and resilience. With each exhalation your mind will become more relaxed, and your body stronger.

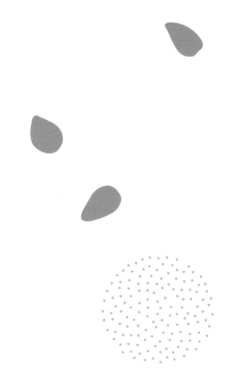

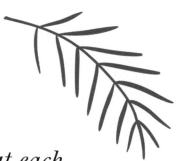

Tell yourself that each breath in brings with it strength and resilience. With each exhalation your mind will become more relaxed, and your body stronger

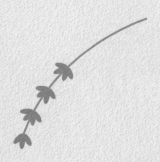

A PREGNANCY PICK-ME-UP

Many expectant mothers find that the tub comes into its own as their pregnancy proceeds and they carry a greater and greater load. Not only does the water take the weight off the feet, hips, and back, a relaxing bath also reduces the stresses and worries that pregnancy naturally prompts—and gives you a precious moment to chat to your bump and bond with the growing baby within.

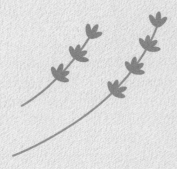

For a full range of specific remedies for pregnancy-related conditions like edema, stretch marks, and morning sickness, you should consult a more detailed resource like Valerie Ann Worwood's *The Fragrant Pharmacy*. This mixture of essential oils comes from that book and her remedy for pregnancy-related exhaustion—it will help you relax, and works as a general pick-me-up for the second or third trimesters.

AROMAS & OILS

Equal amounts of Lavender, Grapefruit, and Coriander combine in a synergistic blend in which each oil complements and amplifies the effects of the others. Grapefruit lowers blood pressure and reduces stress; Coriander will help you sleep; and Lavender calms.

Lavender – 2 drops
Grapefruit – 2 drops
Coriander – 2 drops

Be careful not to overdo the quantity: your body will be more sensitive to essential oils' effects than usual. →

Important: Online, you'll find a host of lists—often conflicting—telling you which essential oils are or aren't safe for pregnant women to use, and little in the way of clear research.

Always play it safe, especially if you have a history of miscarriage: check with your physician or midwife, or a qualified aromatherapist, before using aromatherapy in pregnancy, and avoid essential oils altogether in the first trimester of your baby's development.

In particular, don't use the following oils at any stage: Basil, Laurel, Angelica, Clary Sage, Juniper, Thyme, Cumin, Aniseed, Citronella, and Cinnamon.

MEDITATION

The good news is that there is no risk associated with mindfulness in pregnancy, and excellent evidence that it's one of the best things you can do to look after yourself. Indeed, a 2017 study found that focused mindfulness-based childbirth training was better preparation for labor than conventional prenatal education. This guided mindfulness scan is not that kind of formal training, but regular mindfulness practice is known to help anyone deal with pain and stress. So even if you decide to avoid essential oils during your pregnancy, you can still treat yourself to a warm, candlelit bath treatment and a calming mindfulness exercise.

Close your eyes. Breathe deeply and slowly—in through your nose, then out through your mouth. With each breath, feel the oxygen bringing life to your body, and through you to the baby in your womb. As you exhale, feel your relaxation deepen and deepen. Notice how the water warms you, carries your weight, washes on your bump.

Scan up your body from your feet to your head, noticing any itches, aches, and pains, and naming them without judging them. Notice the areas and joints that are carrying extra weight: ankles, knees, hips, and back. Are they tense or tight? See if they will soften. Notice any aches without judging them. Scan your way up your back and around your torso, noticing all the sensations of your pregnancy, naming them, but not judging them. Notice the pressure of the baby's weight and movements.

Stretch the muscles of your legs, point your toes, and then relax. Breathe steadily in through your nose, out through your mouth as you do. Stretch your arms out, clenching your fists, then relax. Gently point your head to the left and then the right, stretching your neck before rolling your head gently around.

Then notice your whole body, present in this moment. Carry on breathing steadily until you are ready to open your eyes again.

SOUNDS

We know that babies can hear music in the womb and respond to it; they also respond positively to the happy hormones that we enjoy when listening to music ourselves. There is even evidence that it helps their brains develop. Many mothers choose classical works with gently pulsing rhythms—Pachelbel's *Canon in D minor* is a favorite, as is Mozart's *Piano Concerto in C major.*

With each breath, feel the oxygen bringing life to your body, and through you to the baby in your womb

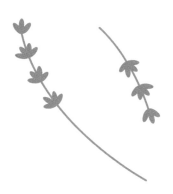

TO WARM UP

There is nothing better than a warm bath to restore you at the end of a cold day. This treatment will get the blood pulsing round your extremities in no time—and help you fight off cold-weather bugs, too.

AROMAS & OILS

Black Pepper will protect you from colds and other opportunistic infections; Marjoram is great for muscle aches and pains; Ginger is profoundly warming and stimulating. Make sure that you have towels or a robe warming for when you get out, then add the drops of essential oil as below and slide gently into the hot water...

Black Pepper – 2 drops
Marjoram – 2 drops
Ginger – 1 drop

MEDITATION

Follow this warming mindful scan and notice as the bath restores you.

Close your eyes. Take deep breaths in through your nose, out through your mouth: count to ten. As you inhale, feel the steamy air of the bathroom restoring you, and as you exhale, feel your relaxation deepen. Notice the water, how it warms you, carries you, presses lightly onto your body.

Notice your feet, their heaviness and lightness, and scan slowly up your body, breathing steadily as you go. Name any aches and pains, any areas of cold, or stiffness, that you come across, but don't judge them. Notice your torso, how it swells and contracts with your breaths, and feel your core returning to the right temperature. If your muscles are tense or tight, let them soften. Breathe steadily in through your nose, out through your mouth, as you go. Stretch and then relax the muscles of your legs, arms, shoulders, and neck. See if they will soften. Notice any pain without judging it.

Scan your whole body until you are completely aware of every sensation. Then notice how present you are in this moment. Breathe steadily until you want to open your eyes again.

SOUNDS

This is a bath that really benefits from slightly more up-tempo music. On a cold day, why not try some hot Southern soul, or seventies' reggae, letting Ken Boothe, Otis Redding, or Candi Staton conjure up a warm summer sun?

TO COOL DOWN

*If you've overheated during the day then a slightly cooler
bath is a great way to restore yourself. Make sure, too, that
you have drunk plenty of water and not become dehydrated.
Obviously, a lower temperature is appropriate here—
100–102 °F (38–39 °C) is around your normal body
temperature, so it will feel neutral. Below that,
the water will actively cool you.*

AROMAS & OILS

Eucalyptus is well known for its
cooling properties, and in this bath is
paired with versatile Lavender, whose
calming properties will restore you to
your natural, balanced temperature.
Check the temperature then add
the essential oils in the following
quantities and step in.

Eucalyptus – 4 drops
Lavender – 4 drops

90

MEDITATION

You may not want to linger in a cool bath once you have returned to a more comfortable temperature, so a long meditation may not be appropriate, but if you are enjoying the water then why not try a simple breathing exercise and mindful body scan?

Close your eyes. Take deep breaths in through your nose, releasing them steadily through your mouth. As you inhale, notice the cool air coming in, and as you exhale, feel heat rushing out. Count ten breaths in and out.

Continuing to breathe slowly, scan up your body, starting with your toes. Notice how the cool water feels around them, and how the muscles and joints relax as you exhale. Scan steadily upwards, checking in with your ankles, calves, knees, and so on. Note and name all of the sensations you feel on your skin and inside your body, but don't judge them or assign them positive or negative qualities.

Continue up through your torso, feeling how your body expands and contracts with each breath. If your chest feels tense or tight, let it soften as you exhale. Breathe steadily in through your nose, out through your mouth, feeling the air flowing into your lungs, filling them as deeply as you can. Notice any itches, aches, and pains, and name them without judging them.

Notice as you cool down to a more comfortable temperature.

Notice the temperature of the water and how it laps against your skin. With each exhalation, relax your muscles, a little more every time. Feel the blood move under your skin, cooling, and taking that coolness back to the core of your body. Carry on breathing deeply and steadily until you're ready to open your eyes once again.

SOUNDS

Obviously, if you're looking to cool down, there's only one serious musical option: cool jazz. So this is the time to dive into Dave Brubeck's *Take Five*, Chet Baker's *Chet Baker Sings*, and Miles Davis' *Birth of the Cool*.

91

A BATH FOR PARENTS

OR CARERS

Lifting, carrying, supporting, putting all of their energy into helping someone else, the carer's lot is not an easy one.

Many feel that they don't have the time or energy to look after themselves. It may seem that way, but taking a moment to look after yourself and restore your strength is incredibly important, ensuring that you can continue to help the person you look after—whether they're your child, your parent, your partner, or anyone in need.

AROMAS & OILS

This mixture combines energy-boosting Orange with regenerating, compassionate Lavender and revitalizing Rosemary. Fill the bath, then when you're ready to step in, add drops in the following proportions:

Orange – 2 drops
Lavender – 3 drops
Rosemary – 1 drop

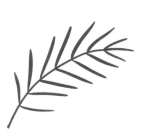

MEDITATION

It's important that you take this opportunity to focus on your own needs and, for a short time, to put those of other people to one side. This is the part of your day when you're putting yourself first: don't feel guilty about that—you need it—and after recharging your own batteries you'll also find that you have more energy and positivity to bring to your caring responsibilities.

So this mindful meditation is all about you, and being in your moment.

Close your eyes. Take several deep breaths in through your nose, releasing them steadily through your mouth. When you inhale, feel the →

Caring responsibilities are usually long term, so if you find this blend works for you, make a candle with it, or a diffuser blend. That way, you'll always have access to a quick aromatherapy hit whenever you need a little support.

fresh oxygen bringing energy to your body, and as you exhale, feel your muscles relaxing ever more deeply in waves from your chest downwards. Count ten breaths in and out.

Continuing to breathe slowly, scan up your body, starting at the soles of your feet. Notice how they feel, and how the muscles and joints relax as you exhale. Track steadily upwards, checking in with your joints, muscles, and skin. Note and name all of the sensations you can feel, without judging them or assigning them positive or negative qualities.

Continue up through your torso, listening to your breath and feeling your body shift as you take in air

and release it. If your chest feels tense or tight, let it soften as you exhale.

Breathe steadily in through your nose, out through your mouth, feeling the air flowing into your lungs, filling them as deeply as you can. Notice any itches, aches, and pains, and name them without judging them. Feel how the bathwater takes some of the weight of your body. Listen for noises in the background, indoors and outdoors, and name the sounds you hear without judging them. Notice the temperature of the water and how it moves against your skin. With each exhalation, relax your muscles, a little more every time.

Carry on breathing deeply and steadily until you are ready to open your eyes once again.

It's important that you take this opportunity to focus on your own needs and, for a short time, to put those of other people to one side

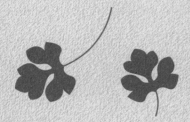

A BATH FOR BETTER DIGESTION

Pain in our stomach or digestive tract can be caused by anything from overeating to anxiety and stress, and it can feel absolutely horrible. If you persistently suffer from indigestion, you should seek medical advice, but if you already know the underlying cause, or if it only strikes occasionally, then this bath will help alleviate the pain and get your digestion working steadily once again.

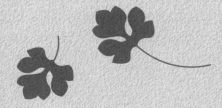

AROMAS & OILS

Many of the most potent essential oils for indigestion are already common in food and drink. This bath uses a warming, heady mixture of Black Pepper, Coriander, Cardamom, and Ginger, which will soothe and relax your aching midriff. When the bath is run, add the oils as below, stretch your arms and torso a couple of times to loosen them, and lower yourself in, submerging yourself in the warm water.

Black Pepper – 2 drops
Coriander – 2 drops
Cardamom – 3 drops
Ginger – 1 drop

MEDITATION

While the essential oils work their magic, this mindful meditation, focused on your torso, will help you deal with the pain and, at the same time, encourage your digestive tract to relax and settle into a more productive rhythm.

Close your eyes. Begin as usual by guiding and paying attention to your breaths: inhale through your nose for one second, hold your breath for a moment, then exhale through your mouth for five seconds or longer. Do this about ten times, counting as you inhale, noticing the flow of air through your mouth and nose and the unique characteristics of each breath.

Carry on breathing steadily, and scan your way up your body, noticing first how your feet and legs feel. Don't rush, work up through your body, and when you come to your torso, and the area that hurts, pay attention to every sensation, painful or not. Observe and name every feeling, but don't judge or react emotionally. With each exhalation, feel the muscles in your torso and abdomen relax: breathe and relax in a flowing rhythm.

Continue to scan through your shoulders and arms to your fingertips and the top of your head. Notice how your body feels, but don't judge.

Now notice the sounds around you, indoors and outdoors, the temperature of the air, the fragrance of the essential oils. Repeat the opening breathing exercise.

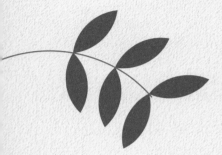
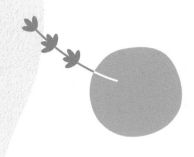

TREATMENTS FOR COMMON AILMENTS

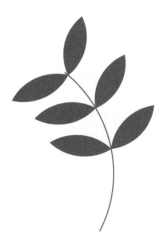

This isn't the place for a complete guide to medical aromatherapy: if you have a more serious ailment that you would like treatment for, then consult a professional or one of the many works of reference available. This short list of treatments for common complaints may give you a starting point, though: it is derived from the work of Rosemary Caddy and Valerie Ann Worwood, whose books are listed on page 140, and which I recommend. Bathing isn't the only way to apply them, of course: depending on the ailment, a lotion, a massage oil, a foot bath, or a diffuser may be appropriate.

Acne: Orange, Cedar, Rosemary, Tea Tree

Athlete's Foot: Lavender, Tea Tree (in a foot bath)

Backache: Chamomile Roman, Eucalyptus, Ginger, Lavender

High Blood Pressure: Clary Sage, Lemon, Ylang Ylang, Lavender, Marjoram

Low Blood Pressure: Thyme, Clove, Cinnamon

Bronchitis: Eucalyptus, Tea Tree, Peppermint, Chamomile Roman

Constipation: Black Pepper, Rosemary, Ginger, Sandalwood

Coughs and Colds: Eucalyptus, Cedarwood, Peppermint

Diarrhea: Ginger, Sandalwood, Chamomile Roman, Geranium

Eczema: Chamomile Roman, Lavender

Headaches: Lavender, Peppermint, Marjoram

Menopause: Clary Sage, Geranium, Lemon (for hot flushes)

Menstrual: Chamomile Roman, Geranium

PMS: Many, depending on symptoms: Nutmeg, Geranium, Bergamot are all particularly effective

Rheumatoid Arthritis: Many, depending on stage and symptoms, but Lavender, Rosemary, Eucalyptus, Chamomile German, Black Pepper, and Clary Sage may be useful

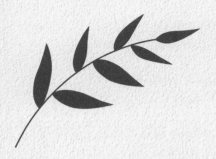

Sometimes, even when we're in good physical health and not facing any particular intellectual challenges, our souls trouble us. We can feel blue for no reason; we can be tortured by anxiety, worry, and stress; or we are simply too tired to feel anything other than flat and unenthusiastic. Alternatively, there may be good external reasons for us to feel sorrow—the loss of a loved one, the end of a relationship, or a career setback.

Whether the root of your emotional problem lies within or not, these simple remedies will help you. Every part of the home spa experience—the water, the aromatherapy, the meditation, the music—has been shown to raise our spirits, and working together they can be a powerful tonic. With a few moments' preparation you can create a nurturing space, from which you'll emerge stronger, more positive, and better equipped to face any of the problems that life brings.

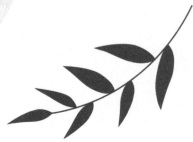

BATHS
for the
SOUL

CHOOSING MUSIC

Music affects our mood.
That's why we listen to it!

But it's not a predictable business: our experience of a song is deeply tied up in our memories, our culture, and our personalities. What moves me most deeply may likely leave you cold, and that's fine. But I think it's possible to make one generalization that everyone can agree with: the most intensely affecting music tends to have powerful vocals. So this is a time to dial up the singers who move you the most deeply. I'm a sucker for old soul belters when I'm feeling emotional, but there's a place here for operatic divas, gospel singers, disco queens, power balladeers, and the great, consoling, spiritual compositions of Bach, Mozart, and Fauré. And don't be shy: join in on the choruses...

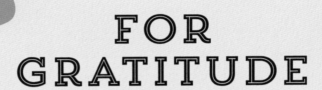

FOR GRATITUDE

We know that gratitude meditation can gently shift our world view, lessening depression, raising feelings of well-being, and even helping us sleep better. Making us more trusting of new people, it can help us deal with challenging social situations, but its benefits are wide and it's no wonder that it has become more and more popular in recent years. In short: gratitude makes you happy.

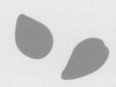

AROMAS & OILS

We should all be grateful for the emotional powers of essential oils! In this blend, Ylang Ylang brings confidence and balance; Frankincense lifts the spirits; Geranium helps to unlock emotions that you may take for granted. When your bath is ready, add the blend below, then take a moment to gratefully anticipate the treatment you're about to enjoy, and step in.

Ylang Ylang – 2 drops
Frankincense – 1 drop
Geranium – 3 drops

If you have time to make one, this blend works well in a candle—a focal point for your meditation.

MEDITATION

Like mindfulness, gratitude meditation is a simple practice with only a few guiding principles. Remember that it works when you not only express gratitude for the good things in your life, but for *everything* in your life. Something that initially seems negative becomes, when you reflect, an opportunity to learn and grow. So recognize the blessings in all things, good, bad, and ugly.

In the bath, shift yourself and shake the tension out of your legs: make yourself completely comfortable. Let your body and mind settle.

Connect with your breathing, slowly inhaling and exhaling. Imagine that with each exhalation you push out tense feelings, and with each inhalation you bring in relaxed feelings to replace them.

Feel this relaxation build in your mind. Notice how your muscles lose tension in the water, watch how the steady breathing brings your heart rate down, and feel your mind and soul relax to match.

It starts at the top of your head, and slowly, warmly, flows down your body. Every time you breathe out, feel your tension dissipate into the air.

When you are relaxed down to your toes, call to mind someone important in your life. Name everything about them that you are grateful for. Recall things that they have done for you, and times that they have been there for you. Be grateful for the times that they have challenged you, too.

Now think gratefully of your home, and name the parts of it that sustain you and bring you joy: the practical aspects, that keep you alive, as well as things that bring you pleasure.

Think of an encounter that you have recently had with someone: positive, negative, or neutral. Reflect gratefully on what it brought you.

Breathing steadily all the time, think of an object or pastime that brings you joy. Express gratitude for how it improves your life. Continue steadily breathing, relaxing, and reflecting for as long as you wish.

FOR JOYFULNESS

Happiness is not just a passive state of mind: it is an activity, too. You can "do" joy, and you will love it!

AROMAS & OILS

This blend of essential oils is upbeat, arousing, positive, and it will spark feelings of happiness, pleasure, and joy in your soul. Seize it! Run with it! Shake the oils into the tub with abandon, then give a little whoop, punch the air, and step in with pleasure!

Sandalwood – 2 drops
Lemon – 2 drops
Bergamot – 2 drops

MEDITATION

This meditation will help you to experience joy in the moment and invite happiness into your life. With regular practice, you will find yourself accessing happy feelings more and more easily, maybe finding that you can "tune in" to them without having to consciously recall happy memories.

Become aware of your breath, slowly breathing in a sense of ease and relaxation. With every breath out, push tension away from your body. Feel the bath warming your body from the outside in, from your skin to your core.

Carry on breathing steadily, relaxing more each time until your muscles are completely loose. Now call to mind a time when you experienced great joy and a sense of well-being. It might be when you were in a beautiful place, or when you had accomplished a personal goal, or when you spent happy moments with a close friend. →

Hold that moment in your mind and recall as much detail as you can. Try to create a picture of it in your mind. What was the place like? Were you there by yourself, or with others? What sensory impressions can you remember—sights, sounds, smells, tastes, textures, or temperature?

Remember how that happiness felt in your mind and body. Did you laugh, smile, jump for joy? Did you feel physically lighter? More energetic? Note how the memory of the moment brings happiness back with it, check in with how that happiness affects your body. Relax into this joyful memory each time you exhale, and notice how that happy memory is now turning this moment into a happy one itself.

Smile, relax, enjoy the moment.

Relax into this joyful memory each time you exhale, and notice how that happy memory is now turning this moment into a happy one itself

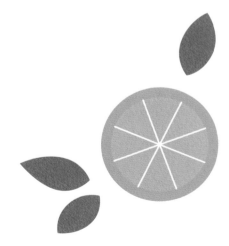

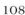

SOUNDS

Right now you want music that triggers the happiest, best memories. So think back to the best concert you ever went to: what was the highlight? What was the moment when you absolutely lost it with excitement and joy? Play that song. Or cast your mind back to a happy night on the dancefloor. What was playing? Use these tunes to drop yourself back into that moment and make the most of this one.

TO RELIEVE STRESS

We've known for thousands of years that bathing relieves stress—that's why so many of us build bathing into our children's bedtime routine. How many times have worn-out parents put a tired, cranky toddler into a warm bath and a few minutes later lifted out a cuddly, sleepy child? This simple treatment will work the same trick, cutting the cortisone from your system, lowering your blood pressure, slowing your heart rate, and in general setting you up for a good night's sleep and a better day tomorrow.

AROMAS & OILS

A host of essential oils have stress-relieving properties, so this is the perfect opportunity to experiment and find out what works for you. This blend is a classic mixture of floral oils: Lavender, Geranium, and Chamomile Roman—all of which have been used for stress relief for generations. There's only a little Lavender in this mixture: more would be overly stimulating. When the bath is ready, stretch your arms out and back, extending them as far as you can, splaying your fingers, and feeling your chest open. Hold your hands above your chest and push your arms back to stretch the shoulders. Then add the oils below to your bath, take one deep breath, exhale, and step in.

Lavender – 1 drop
Geranium – 2 drops
Chamomile Roman – 3 drops

MEDITATION

There are many ways to use meditation to relieve stress. I often use a simple mindfulness scan (like the one on page 77), but a mantra meditation can be effective, too, using the power of repetition to create a profound state of calm as you are lifted out of your distracting train of thought. This one is taken from Tanaaz Chubb's book, *My Pocket Mantras*, and works surprisingly quickly.

Start a rhythm of slow, controlled breathing. Inhale deeply, slowly, steadily, and exhale in the same way. After a few breaths, say the mantra in your mind as you inhale.

With every breath, I feel myself relaxing.

As you finish the mantra, exhale, and notice how your body responds to its message. Repeat, becoming more and more relaxed each time. →

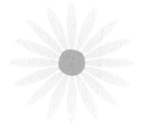

A TENSION-BUSTER

Sometimes, stresses and tensions seem to build up over the course of the day and peak in the evening. You may find that a hard day at work coincides with disagreement at home, or some disappointing news. Maybe there's a simmering difference of opinion in the background that you can't get off your mind? In any case, you need a helping hand. A gratitude meditation is a constructive way to deal with bad news or conflict, while this blend of essential oils will loosen up your muscles. Reducing tension in the body reduces tension in the mind—the beginning of a virtuous circle that will soon have you feeling better.

Anti-inflammatory Eucalyptus here combines with Geranium, a powerful relaxant. Lavender plays its usual role of amplifying the effect of the other oils in the mix. When the bath is ready, shake in the oils as below, and get ready to pass your tension over to the water in the tub...

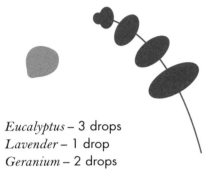

Eucalyptus – 3 drops
Lavender – 1 drop
Geranium – 2 drops

When there's conflict in your life, a gratitude meditation will open your heart and help you to see things from the other point of view. Remember its guiding principle: expressing gratitude not just for the good things in your life, but for *everything* in your life. Challenges, obstacles, and conflict are an opportunity for you to grow, and to become more compassionate.

Make yourself comfortable in the bath. Let your mind and body settle into the water.

Connect with your breath as you inhale and exhale steadily. Imagine that the air you inhale brings relaxation with it, and that the air you exhale takes away tension. Relaxation will build and tension will diminish.

Notice how your muscles relax, observe how steady breaths bring your heart rate right down, and feel relaxation washing down your body from the top of your head to the tips of your toes, flushing away your tension with it.

Now turn your awareness to your surroundings: everything that you can touch, taste, smell, see, and hear. Focus on each object's sensory qualities and say "For this, I am grateful" to each.

Then bring your loved ones to mind: your family, friends, partner, colleagues, even your customers or business partners. Name the things that they bring to your life, and say "For you, I am grateful" to each.

Next, turn to yourself. You are unique! Recognize that you are blessed with a rich imagination, and the ability to communicate and share with others. You can learn from what has passed and plan for what is to come, and you can overcome any difficulties or pain. Name all these attributes, and say "For this, I am grateful" to each.

Finally, reflect on the gift of life. You can learn, grow, share, and work, and enjoy new experiences and sensations without number. Name these possibilities and say "For this, I am grateful" to each.

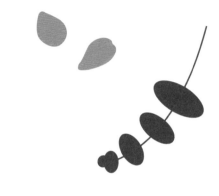

Reducing tension in the body reduces tension in the mind—the beginning of a virtuous circle that will soon have you feeling better

TO REDUCE ANXIETY

Anxiety has a bad reputation, but we need a certain amount of it to survive: it keeps us alert to danger, and stops us from doing reckless things like running over a busy road or eating uncooked meat. But when we start to worry about things we have no control over, or that aren't really so important, it can badly affect our lives. Symptoms can include sleeplessness, headaches, diarrhea, muscle pains, panic attacks, and high blood pressure, and the stress it causes can in turn make us ill. If you feel anxious when you shouldn't, it's time to restore some balance.

Any form of meditation, if you do it regularly, will reduce your levels of anxiety, and you shouldn't wait for the perfect moment—your home spa—if you feel it affecting you. In tough times, I used to retreat to a quiet stairway at the back of the office to calm myself with ten minutes or so of mindfulness. But if you can build it into your everyday routine, then meditation will keep you feeling strong and stable, and you may find that you don't need those emergency sessions anymore.

AROMAS & OILS

If anxiety makes you feel tense, try the treatments on pages 49 and 76. This mixture of essential oils, adapted from Valerie Ann Worwood's book *The Fragrant Mind*, is particularly effective against a more restless, jittery feeling. Cedarwood works on our respiratory system, encouraging calmer breathing; Chamomile Roman quiets the nerves; and Juniper is often used to aid meditation. When the water is ready for you, add these oils to the surface, and step in softly.

Cedarwood – 2 drops
Chamomile Roman – 2 drops
Juniper – 2 drops

MEDITATION

This simple mindfulness scan will help you tune out distracting worries and focus on the moment that you are in.

Close, or half-close, your eyes. Turn your awareness to your breaths in and out, and notice the feeling of water on your skin, and the pressure of your body where it touches the bath.

Breathe steadily, in through your nose and out through your mouth, relaxing every time. Count ten breaths, noting how each is slightly different to the one before.

Then tune in to the sensations in your body: itching, tingling, tension, tightness, or any aches and pains. Scan your way up your body, stopping to note and name—without judgment—any sensations that you come across. Accept every feeling in your body for what it is, then move the focus of your attention onwards. When your attention wanders—as it naturally will—then gently return your attention to your breathing, and how your body feels. Don't reprimand yourself, and don't be frustrated: just steer yourself back on track.

Once you have checked in with every part of your body, turn your attention to the room: the play of candlelight, the fragrance of the bath, the temperature of the water. Notice everything, judge nothing. Be mindfully in the present moment.

FOR GRIEF & LOSS

Grief will happen to all of us: everyone will suffer loss and sorrow, and at some point we lose those whom we love the most, and without whom life barely seems worth living. Creating an atmosphere of acceptance and calm, this bath will help you acknowledge the situation, and start to heal in your own time.

AROMAS & OILS

More than any other oil, Cypress gives us internal strength and helps us bear bad news and live through hard times; it also encourages us to look up, and beyond the everyday. Rose, on the other hand, is comforting and reassuring, expressing the love and affection that we all need. Enlightening Frankincense, finally, will help you move on—even if your steps are, at first, tentative.

Run the bath and add the oils, as follows, before you climb in.

Cypress – 2 drops
Rose – 2 drops
Frankincense – 1 drop

Breathe slowly and deeply in and out through your nose for at least ten minutes.

Many cultures use the flame of a candle to embody our memories of a loved and missed one, and mindfully making your own candle for them might be a constructive way to channel your grief. An extra note of any of the bath's oils could be appropriate: use Frankincense or Cypress if you feel a particular need for strength, and Rose if you need reassurance. Place the candle where you can let your eyes rest on the gentle flame.

MEDITATION

Grief is a natural emotion and, horrible though it is to experience, it will come to us all, and must always be acknowledged: if you attempt to deny or repress feelings of grief or loss, you will only suffer them longer. This meditation is about recognizing the pain without judgment. It goes without saying, though, that if you feel that your grief is unmanageable, you should speak to someone about it: to trusted friends or family, to you or your doctor. →

This aim of this meditation is to allow your emotions to exist without overpowering you. If tears come, that's fine.

Make yourself comfortable in the bath. Notice the places where your body touches it, notice the feeling of water on your skin, and how it supports your weight. Start taking slow, deep breaths, counting one on the inhalations and two on the exhalations.

As you breathe, let the focus of your eyes soften, then feel them become heavy, then close. Turn your attention to your body, and check in with it from top to bottom. Name the sensations that you feel, but don't judge them good or bad.

Notice how each exhalation makes you slightly heavier. Keep your attention gently on the one–two rhythm of your breaths.

Thoughts and feelings will come to mind, quite naturally. When they do, notice them and name them: allow them to exist, without judgment, but always maintain your breathing.

Stay in this state with regular breaths and an awareness of where you are in the moment. Experience every unique breath.

Then let your thoughts wander freely. Let feelings of sadness and loss arise, naturally, and name them as they do, without judging yourself.

Turn your attention back to the body. Notice how your steady breathing has relaxed it and reduced the tension in your muscles.

Notice that you feel lighter. You are still carrying a load, but you know it is manageable, and you are free to acknowledge it to yourself and others.

Notice that you feel lighter. You are still carrying a load, but you know it is manageable, and you are free to acknowledge it to yourself and others

TO BUILD ENTHUSIASM

Enthusiasm makes us extremely attractive, and gives us the energy to take on difficult challenges, too. If you need to bolster yourself before a social occasion like a party or a conference, this bath will boost your self-confidence and energy, so that you can be your best self and light up the room as you walk in. It will also work if you need to recharge yourself to take on a personal task, or a boring job that you've been putting off!

AROMAS & OILS

This trio of oils from citrus fruits has an upbeat fragrance and plenty of get-up-and-go. Grapefruit refreshes and revives; Lemon clears and energizes the mind; Orange is joyful and uplifting. You'll hop out of this bath with a smile on your face! When the water is ready for you, add the oils in the proportions below, and inhale the citrus scents as they rise from it. Then step in.

Grapefruit – 2 drops
Lemon – 2 drops
Orange – 2 drops

MEDITATION

This visualizing meditation will prepare you well for a specific challenge—or simply give you a boost and lift your spirits.

Take steady, deep breaths, counting them as you go: breathe evenly in through your nose and out through your mouth. Focus on the air moving in and out, and notice the details in each breath. Take at least ten breaths like this, and feel yourself relaxing further with each one. →

SOUNDS

In this state, almost any music should sound good! One good way to celebrate it would be to find a performance in which an artist enjoys and celebrates their own skills. Pick a tune with whoops and hollers and *joie de vivre*—maybe a live take with plenty of audience noise, or a song with a jaw-dropping solo. This is the right bath for some air guitar!

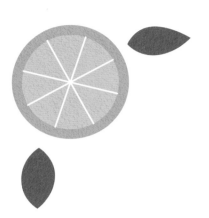

Then start to check in with your body, scanning it from top to bottom so that you are absolutely in the moment. Note how every part of your body feels: identify itches, aches, pains, places that are stiff—but don't judge them. Focus on relaxing with each breath out.

Now ask yourself what you want to accomplish. Name it, without judgment. What do you not want to do? Name that, too, without judging yourself.

Think back to a day when you accomplished a similar goal, a day when everything went your way. Name the emotions that you felt, and the things that you did.

Feel the energy levels rise in your body as you remember that success.

Now visualize the task ahead of you: imagine yourself as you will be, whether that's socializing or working. See yourself succeeding, and accomplishing what you need to do.

Picture yourself making the right choices, staying focused on your role, and making strong connections with other people.

Take the positive energy from this moment and see yourself applying it to your challenge.

See yourself doing it all with a smile on your face, energetic and confident: standing tall, making eye contact with people, radiating positive energy, kindness, and confidence.

Feel yourself embodying this enthusiasm.

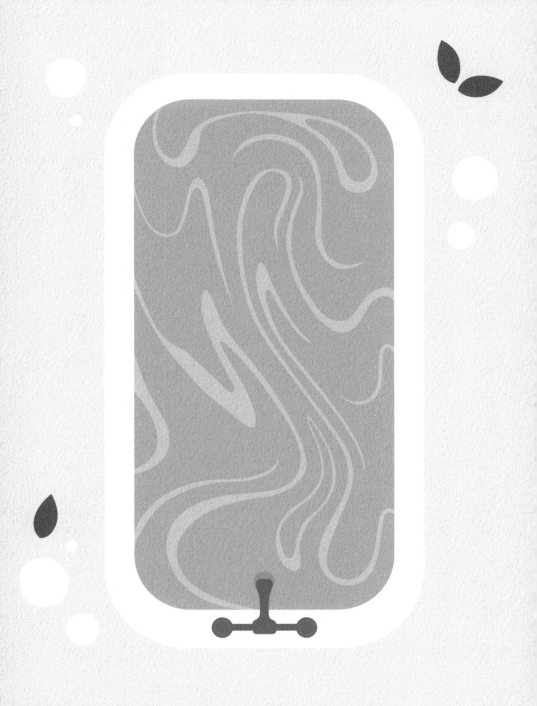

TO REDUCE ANGER

Of all the baths in this book, this is the one that has done me the most good. I don't get angry often, but if I do, and I'm at home, the first thing I do is grab a towel and head for the bathroom for half an hour. With a clear, cool head, it's always easier to process whatever it was you got angry about, take that angry energy, point it in a positive direction, and move on with your life.

AROMAS & OILS

All three of these oils will help you let go of angry feelings and find peace: if you have Chamomile German, that will work instead of Chamomile Roman. Any Rose oil (Absolute, Maroc, or Otto) should be effective. Lavender calms and restores balance; Chamomile reduces tension; Rose opens your heart and helps you understand other points of view. When the bath is run, add the oils in the proportions below, take a deep breath, step in, and simmer down...

Chamomile Roman – 3 drops
Lavender – 2 drops
Rose – 2 drops

MEDITATION

Meditation is an effective way to address and let go of anger, but you have to want it to work, so you may not immediately be in the right frame of mind. If, when you climb into the bath, your heart is still pounding and your adrenalin is running high, then give the essential oils a few minutes to work their magic, and concentrate on the breathing exercises before embarking on the meditation proper.

Take steady, deep breaths, counting each one: breathe steadily in through the nose and out through the mouth. Focus on the air moving in and out, notice the details in each breath, and how the rate of breathing slows slightly as you calm down. With each exhalation, relax your body. Breathe this way until you feel your anger subsiding.

SOUNDS

Something calm and considered, perhaps low-tempo and philosophical in feel. A spot of Leonard Cohen or Joni Mitchell?

Make sure that your hands are open, not clenched. Then check in with your body, scanning it from top to bottom. Note how every part of your body feels: identify physical sensations, but don't judge them. If you feel your attention drifting away, or returning to your feelings of anger, gently return your thoughts to your scan. Relax with each breath out.

Continue to breathe, feeling the tension diminish with every out breath.

Recognize any anger that remains: don't judge it, don't make it positive or negative, think of it as a pot of boiling water on the stove, neither good nor bad in itself. As you visualize the pot, think of yourself turning down the heat, and watch the water stop boiling, and start to cool.

Think of your anger cooling with every breath you take outwards.

Continue to focus on your breathing, and relaxing your body, and visualizing the pot as it cools right down. Stay in the bath until your anger has subsided and been replaced by calmer feelings.

FOR HEARTBREAK

We are told that time is the best cure for a
broken heart, and there is some truth to that.
But time passes slowly, and we can help ourselves
get over the pain of heartbreak more quickly if
we consciously put our feelings into perspective.
This treatment will help you step back, and
value what's really important.

AROMAS & OILS

These oils will all work on your heart, helping it to heal and reducing the pain of your broken relationship. They will also help you deal with feelings of loss and loneliness. Rose Otto opens your heart and helps with loneliness; Chamomile Roman is soothing and comforting; Lavender helps with low mood; and Bergamot, one of the most positive oils, lifts the heart.

This powerful remedy is well suited to the pain of heartbreak: when your bath is ready, add the oils in the proportions below, and step into the supportive water.

Rose Otto – 3 drops
Chamomile Roman – 2 drops
Lavender – 2 drops
Bergamot – 2 drops

MEDITATION

When you name your painful emotions, you remove much of their destructive power. This meditation will guide you to calmly examine your feelings, giving them compassionate attention and noticing them without judging.

Start by controlling your breathing, in and out: notice each inhalation, each exhalation. If it helps, count your breaths. In any case, pay attention to each one, feeling how different every breath is to the one before.

With each exhalation, feel your whole body relaxing.

Now scan your body from your head to your toes: notice and name every sensation you can feel, every ache, itch, tightness. Don't judge them, merely note them, explore them, and move on to the next. Let your body relax each time you breathe out.

When your body is relaxed, imagine that with each breath you inhale the future, and exhale the past. Picture yourself moving forwards, drawn on by each inhalation.

If you feel the pain of heartbreak, treat it as you treated aches and itches a moment ago. Pay attention to it, name it, but do not judge it. Instead, with gentle curiosity, notice its components. Is there pain, loneliness, or guilt? Are you angry with yourself, or the other person, or someone else? Do you feel unfairly treated, or rejected, or unlovable? Notice all of these feelings and name them.

Now you have named the elements of your heartbreak, consider that they are all stepping stones as you move forwards. The relationship that is over is a part of your past, steps on your journey—but not your destination. Reflect on what the relationship taught you, and how you can use that knowledge in the next chapter of your life.

Call to mind the other person in the relationship, thank them for what you learned from the time you shared, and let them go.

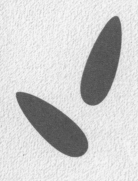

AWAY FROM HOME

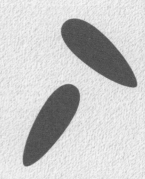

Whether you're traveling for business or pleasure, a hotel room can be a lonely, alienating place. Far from your loved ones, it's possible to feel overwhelmed by jet lag, homesickness, loneliness, or worries that you would normally take in your stride. But there is usually an upside—a nice clean tub, and a stack of crisp towels. So before you travel, prepare a dose of this remedy, which will help you adjust to your new surroundings, appreciate them, and enjoy a good night's sleep. By reminding you of home at the most basic level—scents—it will bring you deep feelings of comfort and security, and help you sleep.

MUSIC FOR TRAVELERS

You can surprise yourself with some local music—songs from this unfamiliar town or country, which will give you a deeper connection to it—or you can bring a little bit of home with you. Listen to the favorite songs of the people you miss, or make a nostalgic selection and indulge in a little sentimental homesickness.

AROMAS & OILS

Clary Sage will help counter any melancholy worries, and will ground you in your new surroundings; Marjoram will bolster your courage and perseverance; versatile Lavender will pull them together and add a floral note of peace and restfulness. Balance them as seems best to you, or use the ratio below. Add them when the bath is full, and step in.

Clary Sage – 2 drops
Marjoram – 1 drop
Lavender – 2 drops

MEDITATION

Begin as usual by noticing the life-giving air that flows in and out of your body: inhale through your nose for a second, hold your breath for two seconds, then exhale over five seconds or more. Repeat this ten times, noticing the flow of air through your mouth and nose, the movements of your chest as you inhale and exhale, and the fact that every breath is slightly different from the one before.

With your eyes closed, carry on breathing steadily and meditatively, and work your way up your body, checking in with the feet that brought you here, your legs, your torso, and so on: tense up, then relax the muscles in each area, and notice how they feel. Thank each limb in turn for bringing you safely to this new place.

Now open your eyes and notice your unfamiliar surroundings. Without judging any part of it, let your eyes wander all over this strange room that will be yours for a short time. Notice the background hum of life going on in the hotel, and identify individual sounds if you can.

Still breathing steadily, make yourself present in your temporary home. Take a part of it into you, and leave a part of yourself there.

Your hotel may not allow you to burn candles in the bathroom; think ahead and prepare a homemade bubble bath or bath oil before your travels.

TO HEAD OFF PANIC

Panic attacks are one of the most terrible manifestations of anxiety and fear. When one strikes, it feels like your world is caving in uncontrollably, and it's certainly not possible to calm down enough to have a relaxing home spa treatment. Concentrate on your breathing, change the scene, and let it subside. There is, fortunately, always some kind of calm after the storm, and this is when you should take action to make sure that you don't suffer another one.

The first, most important, step is to seek professional advice and help, and follow the advice that you receive. There may be a medical, or biological, cause for the attacks. But if the cause is accumulated worry, stress, anxiety, or loss, there are simple things that you can do yourself to lower the risk of any return.

You should look after your mind, and regularly allow your emotions and fears a safe outlet: this treatment will give you a space to do that. Make time to do it regularly.

AROMAS & OILS

Bergamot oil calms and reduces agitation. Some people find that Orange reduces fear of the unknown—often a component in panic disorders—and it also brings optimism. Rose Otto is one of the most powerful essential oils for the soul, reducing anxiety and strengthening our spirit. When the water is ready, add the oils in the proportions below, and step into your oasis of calm.

Bergamot – 3 drops
Orange – 2 drops
Rose Otto – 2 drops

MEDITATION

This meditation should create a safe time and space for your emotions to well up so that you can identify them and, in doing so, reduce their destructive powers. Many panic attacks are caused by fears that we have not properly acknowledged, and simply naming them will help.

Relax into the moment. Stretch and shake out your limbs so that you are comfortable, and note how the water feels.

Start by controlling your breathing and attend to every inhalation, every exhalation. If it helps, count your breaths with a one–two rhythm. Pay attention to each, and notice how unique each breath is.

With each exhalation, feel your whole body relax and become slightly looser, slightly heavier.

Now scan your body from head to toe: notice and name every sensation you feel, every ache, itch, tightness. Don't judge, merely note them, explore them, name them, and move on. When you are at one with the

moment, let your mind wander. As thoughts and emotions arise, check in with them, and name them, but don't judge them.

As you notice fears or worries, treat them as you just treated the sensations in your body. Pay attention to them, name them, and with gentle curiosity, notice their components. What do you fear? What worries you? Is there vulnerability, or helplessness? Notice all your feelings and name them.

Continue to breathe steadily, and once you have acknowledged each rising thought or emotion, gently turn your attention back to your breathing.

Remain in the water while the meditation comes to a natural end, then lie there and enjoy your moment of calm. When you get out, resolve to carry the positive effects of the treatment with you.

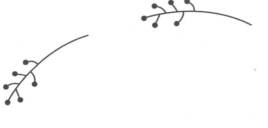

*Many panic attacks
are caused by fears that
we have not properly
acknowledged, and simply
naming them will help*

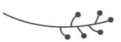

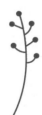

A BATH FOR CONFIDENCE

If you don't feel confident about a specific challenge that's ahead of you, then try the Mental Energy Boost on page 40. If, however, you persistently suffer from a lack of confidence, then try to follow this treatment regularly.

AROMAS & OILS

Cardamom is grounding and fortifying, as well as positive; optimistic Grapefruit lifts self-esteem; and Jasmine is known to bring confidence, warmth, and positivity. When the tub is full, shake these oils onto the surface of the bathwater, then sink into the welcoming, sustaining water.

Cardamom – 2 drops
Grapefruit – 3 drops
Jasmine – 2 drops

MEDITATION

Shake and stretch out your limbs so they are comfortable, then lie back in the bath. Place the palm of your right hand over your breastbone and the palm of your left hand over your navel.

Breathe slowly and deeply, feeling your chest rise and fall as you do so. As you inhale, count one as you exhale, then count two, feeling your body relax more with each exhalation. Let your eyes gradually close as you continue focused breathing for a minute or two.

Notice the strength and power of your breath through the palms of your hands. Feel the power of your diaphragm, the muscle that controls your breathing and that is always there for you, reliably keeping you going, every moment of every day.

Witness your thoughts as they rise into your consciousness, and notice what they are, but don't judge them. Identify any thoughts that are self-limiting, or unconfident, and name them as such—but don't judge them, or yourself.

Now replace those thoughts, saying to yourself, "I have done difficult things before, and I can do them again," or, if more appropriate, "I know a lot, and I can learn even more." Repeat this line gently, as a mantra, with the first part of the line on an inhalation and the second part on an exhalation.

Feel your body filling with belief and confidence. Picture it running to the end of every fingertip.

Continue to breathe steadily and deeply to nourish this confidence.

A SPA TREATMENT FOR MOOD SWINGS

Mood swings are difficult to live with, and they can make us difficult to live with, too. Meditation, with its powerful grounding effects, is undoubtedly one of the best things that anyone can do to limit their unpredictable ups and downs. If you can make this a regular part of your routine, and then combine it with a balancing aromatherapy treatment, so much the better.

AROMAS & OILS

Geranium counteracts excesses of emotions with balance and harmony; Cardamom grounds us; Cedarwood brings fortitude, reliability, and steadiness. Add the drops as directed below, have a stretch and a shake of the limbs, then step into the water.

Geranium – 3 drops
Cardamom – 3 drops
Cedarwood – 3 drops

MEDITATION

Start by observing your breaths. Give them your full attention—counting them may help you stay focused—inhaling slowly through your nose, and exhaling through your mouth. Witness how each breath slightly differs from the one before, and register how deep, long, and steady each one is.

Now scan your body from the head down, noting all the sensations you find—discomforts, itches, aches, where you feel the water or the tub. Name every sensation, but don't judge anything. Feel yourself becoming more relaxed with every exhalation.

If your attention wanders at any point, gently return it to scanning and breathing.

When you are completely relaxed and present in the moment, let thoughts and emotions naturally arise. Watch them, and name them, without judging: they may be happy or sad, positive or negative. Notice what prompts each thought, what lies beneath it, but don't judge them or yourself.

Let your mind wander, observing thoughts as they come and go. Return your attention to your breaths. With each exhalation, feel your body and mind become more relaxed. As they stay in this slow rhythm, imagine that each breath in brings balance, and each breath out carries away instability and volatility.

137

A BATH FOR A LOVER (OR LOVERS...)

There is no better way to prepare yourself for the physical expression of love than a warm candlelit bath, laden with aphrodisiacs. Collect yourself, enjoy the moment of anticipation, and maybe invite someone in to share it with you?

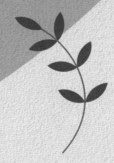

AROMAS & OILS

Many oils are reputed to have sensual, aphrodisiac qualities, including Bergamot, Rose Otto, Neroli, Melissa, Cardamom, Sandalwood, Clary Sage, Frankincense, and Jasmine. This blend should not disappoint… And it's all about pleasure. So when you've added these heady oils to the full bath, take a moment to inhale their vapors, then slowly slide into the hot water...

Sandalwood – 3 drops
Jasmine – 3 drops
Bergamot – 3 drops

MEDITATION

All of the usual benefits of mindfulness meditation—higher energy, lower stress, more empathy, more self-confidence—are, of course, highly sexy. This exercise will make you completely present in the moment, which you and your partner will definitely enjoy.

Focus on your breathing with a one–two rhythm. Count one on each deep inhalation through your nose, and two on each exhalation through your mouth. Let yourself relax; feel the inhalations carrying in energy, and the exhalations taking out stress and tiredness.

Become aware of each one of your senses in turn:

Sound—name all the sounds you can hear in this moment.

Sight—observe the quality of the light in the room, reflections on the water, and the play of shadows.

Smell—identify the fragrances of your essential oils, your own body, and anything else in the room.

Taste—pay attention to your tongue and mouth, naming any tastes you can identify.

Touch—feel where your body touches the bath, the pressure of your weight, and the weight of the water. Notice how the water feels on your skin.

Return your attention to your breath and feel each one carrying currents of energy passing around your body. With each exhalation, feel your skin become more sensitive, your senses more receptive, and the energy levels rising ever higher.

REFERENCES & FURTHER READING

AROMATHERAPY

In writing this book I have drawn heavily on two books in particular: *The Fragrant Pharmacy* and *The Fragrant Mind*, both by Valerie Ann Worwood. Both are strongly recommended to anyone who wants to go deeper into the amazing art of essential oils. *The Essential Blending Guide* by Rosemary Caddy is excellent on the constituent molecules that give essential oils their remarkable powers. I've also referred extensively to *Aromatherapy: A Nurse's Guide* by Ann Percival, *Aromatherapy: A Guide for Home Use* by Christine Westwood, and *The Aromatherapy Bible* by Gill Farrer-Halls.

MINDFULNESS & MEDITATION

The internet is a wonderful resource for anyone interested in exploring mindfulness or meditation in general. Your first stop should be Mindful.Org, which has plenty to help you develop in mindfulness meditation; several of the exercises in this book are adapted from ones on their site. In addition, I've referred to meditations on the following sites—in many cases, I've practiced them myself—and I encourage you to check them out. There are also untold thousands of meditations on YouTube: you will easily find a channel with sessions that are right for you.

www.headspace.com
www.health.harvard.edu
www.northshore.org
www.unchainmybrain.com
www.ananda.com
www.jameshollis.net
www.mindfulliving.coach
www.insighttimer.com/christina sianmcmahon
www.alignedandwell.com
www.positivepsychology.com
www.happify.com
www.lamaze.org
www.mindworks.com
www.verywellmind.com

INDEX

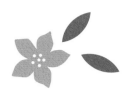

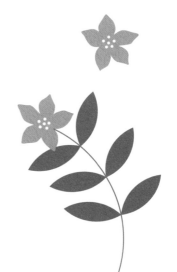

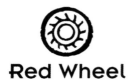

Red Wheel

This edition first published in 2022 by Red Wheel Books, an imprint of
Red Wheel/Weiser, LLC
With offices at:
65 Parker Street, Suite 7
Newburyport, MA 01950
www.redwheelweiser.com

ISBN: 978-1-59003-533-7
Library of Congress Cataloging-in-Publication Data available upon request.

Cover design by Red Wheel/Weiser
Cover illustration by Louise Evans
Interior illustrations and design by Louise Evans
Printed by PNB in Latvia

10 9 8 7 6 5 4 3 2 1

MIX
Paper from
responsible sources
FSC™ C007454
FSC
www.fsc.org